UROLOGY RESEARCH PROGRESS

T0293027

URINARY INCONTINENCE

PREVALENCE, RISK FACTORS AND MANAGEMENT STRATEGIES

UROLOGY RESEARCH PROGRESS

Additional books in this series can be found on Nova's website
under the Series tab.

Additional e-books in this series can be found on Nova's website
under the e-book tab.

UROLOGY RESEARCH PROGRESS

URINARY INCONTINENCE

PREVALENCE, RISK FACTORS AND MANAGEMENT STRATEGIES

DEBRA NEWTON
EDITOR

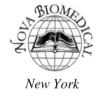

New York

Copyright © 2016 by Nova Science Publishers, Inc.

NOTICE TO THE READER

Library of Congress Cataloging-in-Publication Data

ISBN: 978-1-53610-099-0
Library of Congress Control Number: 2016951321

Published by Nova Science Publishers, Inc. † New York

CONTENTS

PREFACE

Urinary incontinence (UI) is defined as the complaint of involuntary loss of urine. Urinary incontinence can be divided into several different types, including stress urinary incontinence (SUI), which is defined as the complaint of involuntary loss of urine on effort, physical exertion, sneezing or coughing. Mixed urinary incontinence (MUI) is defined as the complaint of involuntary leakage associated with urgency and effort, exertion, sneezing and coughing. Urge urinary incontinence (UUI) is defined as the complaint of involuntary leakage accompanied by or immediately preceded by urgency; overflow incontinence, and functional incontinence. This book reviews UI's prevalence, risk factors and the management strategies currently available.

Chapter 1 - Urinary incontinence (UI), defined as the complaint of involuntary loss of urine, is a common condition among women during pregnancy and the postpartum period. UI can be divided into several different types, including stress urinary incontinence (SUI), mixed urinary incontinence (MUI), urge urinary incontinence (UUI), overflow incontinence and functional incontinence. However, SUI, MUI and UUI are the most common types of UI among pregnant and postpartum women. The most common type of urinary incontinence (UI) in pregnant women is SUI, followed by MUI and UUI.

Pregnancy may also be associated with reduced pelvic floor muscle (PFM) strength, which can cause UI. Both physiological and hormonal changes during pregnancy may lead to disruption in the normal urinary tract function and weaken the supportive and sphincteric function of PFM. Hence, when intra-abdominal pressure increases, the urethral sphincter is not strong enough to close the urethra, thereby resulting in urine leakage.

The prevalence of UI varies depending on the use of different populations, study designs, methods for assessing incontinence, definitions of UI, evaluation questionnaires, stage of pregnancy and duration following childbirth. The prevalence of UI during pregnancy is estimated to range from 10.8% to 84.12%. The prevalence of UI also increases with gestational age and peaks during the third trimester of pregnancy. SUI is the most common type of UI during pregnancy, and the overall prevalence rate of SUI (4% to 78.8%) is higher than MUI (13.1% to 24.8%) and UUI (5.9% to 12.9%).

The prevalence of UI reaches a maximum during pregnancy and decreases after childbirth. During the postpartum period, the overall prevalence of postpartum UI ranges from 2.7% to 76.4% with a remission rate of three months after childbirth of up to 86.4%. The most common type of UI in postpartum women is SUI (5.0% to 57%), followed by MUI (47.5%) and UUI (5.5% to 44.0%).

UI can affect the psychological and social well-being of women. UI can also have long-term effects on quality of life (QOL) and is associated with enormous health-related costs. UI is known to have detrimental effects on QOL in approximately 54.3% of pregnant women. Pregnant women with UI have statistically significant lower QOL during pregnancy than those without UI, and the QOL of incontinent pregnant women worsens with increasing gestational age to term. Moreover, pregnant women with UUI or MUI have worse QOL scores during pregnancy than those with SUI alone.

UI not only affects QOL during pregnancy, but also affects QOL during the postpartum period. Therefore, UI is a serious health problem during the postpartum period and affects the QOL of postpartum women by disrupting daily activities. Postpartum women who have UI are associated with feelings of frustration and embarrassment. Approximately three-fourths (74%) of postpartum women with UI report mild UI, and 26% of these report moderate UI, while none report severe UI. The prevalence of depressive symptoms is higher in women with UI than in those without UI.

The purpose of this chapter on the presentation of data from several studies of UI in pregnant and postpartum women is to review and discuss the prevalence, types and severity of UI among women from pregnancy to the postpartum period. Understanding these issues can be useful for healthcare professionals in delivering more informed counseling to women to help prevent UI during pregnancy and the postpartum period.

Chapter 2 - Urinary incontinence (UI), the complaint of involuntary loss of urine, is a common condition during the immediate postpartum period after a woman's first pregnancy. The prevalence of UI is high and approximately 18.96% to 55.9% of all pregnant women develop UI during pregnancy. During the postpartum period, the prevalence of UI ranges from 6.9% to 47.0%, which is lower when compared with the prevalence during the third trimester of pregnancy. However the remission rate of UI at three months after childbirth as high as 86.4%.

UI is a serious health problem during the postpartum period that affects the quality of life (QoL) of postpartum women by disrupting the women's daily activities. Postpartum women who have UI feel frustrated and embarrassed.

It is well known that UI is related to the weakening of the pelvic floor muscle (PFM), connective tissue and fascia as well as their supportive and sphincteric function. The pathophysiology of UI is multifactorial but there is a lot of evidence to support the critical role of pregnancy and vaginal delivery in the development of UI. Pregnancy may be associated with a reduction in PFM strength that can develop into UI. In addition to pregnancy itself, the physiological changes associated with the second stage of labor can cause significant stress on the PFM appear to play a role in postpartum UI. However, the exact causes of postpartum UI remain unclear.

Several risk factors have been proven to be associated with UI, some of which are potentially modifiable to facilitate early intervention for target at risk women. Aging is an important role in UI development in the form of genetic risk factors. The other significant modifiable risk factors for postpartum UI include high body mass index, obesity, smoking, constipation, multiparity, UI before pregnancy, UI during pregnancy, prolonged second stage of labor, mode of delivery and neonatal birth weight. Antenatal UI increases the risk for postpartum incontinence, which in turn increases the risk for long–term persistent UI. The second stage of labor has modest effects on postpartum PFM function. After their first delivery, women who deliver vaginally have a higher incidence of postpartum SUI than those who deliver by cesarean section (C/S). Postpartum women who have higher BMI and weight retention at six months postpartum are at increased risk for postpartum UI.

In decreasing the risk for postpartum UI, pregnant women who perform pelvic floor muscle exercises (PFME) may be able to prevent postpartum UI. Postpartum weight loss by advice about eating and exercise habits to avoid weight retention after delivery can also decrease the risk for UI and restore the continence mechanism at six months postpartum. Moreover, elective cesarean sections in these women also have a preventive effect and lower the risk for developing postpartum UI.

The purpose of this review chapter is to identify the risk factors for the development of UI in postpartum women. This understanding can be useful for health professionals in educating and counseling pregnant and postpartum women about preventing and reducing the risk factors contributing to the development of UI during postpartum period.

Chapter 3 - Urinary incontinence (UI), the complaint of involuntary loss of urine, is a common condition among women in various population ages, which has significant impact on quality of life (QoL). Estimates of the prevalence of UI vary greatly with reports ranging from approximately 2.7% to 84.12% of all women in population ages.

UI affects the QoL of women in four domains including physical activity, travel, social relationships and emotional health. Several incontinent women have responded that UI restricts lifestyles, inhibits daily activities, interferes with social activities and sexual function, and results in a loss of self-confidence. Specifically, several women who had UI symptoms have reported that UI decreases overall QoL with feelings of embarrassment, depression, anxiety, difficulty and discomfort. More than half (60%) of the women reported that they suffered moderate to extreme discomfort or difficulty caused by their UI symptoms.

The predicting factors of treatment-seeking behavior among incontinent women are associated with various factors such as older age, long duration and greater severity of UI symptoms with higher emotional and physical impact on QoL, more discomfort and perceived UI suffering. Women suffering from severe UI are significantly more likely to have sought treatment than those with mild to moderate UI. Therefore, the major reasons for treatment-seeking are perceived increase in severity or distress and the need for incontinence materials. In many countries, women with UI who have treatment-seeking behavior can directly visit general practitioners (GP), specialists, gynecologists or urologists to consult about their UI symptoms. However, the rate of treatment-seeking for UI is significantly lower when compared to UI prevalence. The rate of treatment-seeking behavior among incontinent women is reported at approximately 15% to 45%.

The barrier factors of treatment-seeking behavior among UI women are also associated with various factors including older age, different racial and ethnic groups, social stigmas, embarrassment about visiting healthcare providers, consideration of UI as a normal consequence of pregnancy, childbirth or aging, characteristics and types of UI, perception that UI severity is not a serious or life-threatening problem, insufficient knowledge about urinary incontinence and treatment, healthcare professionals or healthcare providers, and other factors such as perceived self-efficacy and counseling about UI symptoms from healthcare providers.

Therefore, several women tend to consider UI as a common problem in women that is inevitable with age, especially in older age. Most women who do not seek treatment do not do so because they consider their incontinence as not a very serious problem, have deficient knowledge about UI etiology and available treatments. The majority of women are not provided with information on UI by health professionals. Moreover, incontinent women who have mild symptoms of UI or do not experience daily leakage and those who do not perceive leakage as a serious troublesome with impact on their daily lives do not want treatment-seeking. The rate of non-treatment-seeking behavior among incontinent women is reported at approximately 50% to 80%. Although these women are often inconvenienced and troubled by UI symptoms, they are reluctant to seek help from health professionals. Moreover, approximately two-thirds of suffering women who do not seek help are too embarrassed to do so.

The purpose of this chapter is to review and discuss the predictive and barrier factors associated with treatment-seeking behavior among women with UI. This information can be useful for healthcare professionals when informing and counseling women who have UI to promote women's knowledge about seeking treatment for urine leakage.

Chapter 4 - Urinary incontinence (UI) is a common disease in elderly women. It is classified into stress UI, urgency UI and mixed UI based on different etiology. It has been recommended that potential benefits and risks should be considered before a therapeutic strategy being developed for patients with UI. Compared to surgery, non-surgical management is more likely to be accepted by patients. Furthermore, more and more evidences have show the efficacy of these non-invasive treatment. In this chapter, the authors will present the evidence about the effectiveness of these treatments, as well as their potential mechanism, on different types of UI. In terms of specific treatment, lifestyle interventions, behavioral and physical therapies, and pharmacological management will be discussed for each type of UI. Besides, the complementary and alternative medicine treatment will also be involved. In particular, the authors will share their clinical experience and present the evidence from their research in management of UI.

In: Urinary Incontinence
Editor: Debra Newton

ISBN: 978-1-53610-099-0
© 2016 Nova Science Publishers, Inc.

Chapter 1

URINARY INCONTINENCE: PREVALENCE, TYPE AND SEVERITY FROM PREGNANCY TO POSTPARTUM

Nucharee Sangsawang[1],*, Bussara Sangsawang[1] and Denchai Laiwattana[2]
[1]Department of Maternal–Child Nursing and Midwifery Nursing, Faculty of Nursing, Srinakharinwirot University, Thailand
[2]Department of Neurosurgery, Bangkok Hospital Trat, Trat, Thailand

ABSTRACT

Urinary incontinence (UI), defined as the complaint of involuntary loss of urine, is a common condition among women during pregnancy and the postpartum period. UI can be divided into several different types, including stress urinary incontinence (SUI), mixed urinary incontinence (MUI), urge urinary incontinence (UUI), overflow incontinence and functional incontinence. However, SUI, MUI and UUI are the most common types of UI among pregnant and postpartum women. The most common type of urinary incontinence (UI) in pregnant women is SUI, followed by MUI and UUI.

Pregnancy may also be associated with reduced pelvic floor muscle (PFM) strength, which can cause UI. Both physiological and hormonal changes during pregnancy may lead to disruption in the normal urinary

---

* Corresponding author: twinnuch-swu@hotmail.com.

tract function and weaken the supportive and sphincteric function of PFM. Hence, when intra-abdominal pressure increases, the urethral sphincter is not strong enough to close the urethra, thereby resulting in urine leakage.

The prevalence of UI varies depending on the use of different populations, study designs, methods for assessing incontinence, definitions of UI, evaluation questionnaires, stage of pregnancy and duration following childbirth. The prevalence of UI during pregnancy is estimated to range from 10.8% to 84.12%. The prevalence of UI also increases with gestational age and peaks during the third trimester of pregnancy. SUI is the most common type of UI during pregnancy, and the overall prevalence rate of SUI (4% to 78.8%) is higher than MUI (13.1% to 24.8%) and UUI (5.9% to 12.9%).

The prevalence of UI reaches a maximum during pregnancy and decreases after childbirth. During the postpartum period, the overall prevalence of postpartum UI ranges from 2.7% to 76.4% with a remission rate of three months after childbirth of up to 86.4%. The most common type of UI in postpartum women is SUI (5.0% to 57%), followed by MUI (47.5%) and UUI (5.5% to 44.0%).

UI can affect the psychological and social well-being of women. UI can also have long-term effects on quality of life (QOL) and is associated with enormous health-related costs. UI is known to have detrimental effects on QOL in approximately 54.3% of pregnant women. Pregnant women with UI have statistically significant lower QOL during pregnancy than those without UI, and the QOL of incontinent pregnant women worsens with increasing gestational age to term. Moreover, pregnant women with UUI or MUI have worse QOL scores during pregnancy than those with SUI alone.

UI not only affects QOL during pregnancy, but also affects QOL during the postpartum period. Therefore, UI is a serious health problem during the postpartum period and affects the QOL of postpartum women by disrupting daily activities. Postpartum women who have UI are associated with feelings of frustration and embarrassment. Approximately three-fourths (74%) of postpartum women with UI report mild UI, and 26% of these report moderate UI, while none report severe UI. The prevalence of depressive symptoms is higher in women with UI than in those without UI.

The purpose of this chapter on the presentation of data from several studies of UI in pregnant and postpartum women is to review and discuss the prevalence, types and severity of UI among women from pregnancy to the postpartum period. Understanding these issues can be useful for healthcare professionals in delivering more informed counseling to women to help prevent UI during pregnancy and the postpartum period.

INTRODUCTION

Urinary incontinence (UI), defined as the complaint of involuntary loss of urine, is a common condition among women during pregnancy and the postpartum period [1]. Urinary incontinence can be divided into several different types, including stress urinary incontinence (SUI), which is defined as the complaint of involuntary loss of urine on effort, physical exertion, sneezing or coughing. Mixed urinary incontinence (MUI) is defined as the complaint of involuntary leakage associated with urgency and effort, exertion, sneezing and coughing. Urge urinary incontinence (UUI) is defined as the complaint of involuntary leakage accompanied by or immediately preceded by urgency; overflow incontinence, and functional incontinence [1].

The pathophysiology of UI is multifactorial and thought to be related to a general weakening of the pelvic floor muscles and the collagen-dependent tissues involved in pelvic support as a result of pregnancy and parturition [2]. Under normal conditions, UI does not occur because of the body's continence mechanism which is dependent on the normal functioning of the lower urinary tract such as the bladder as well as the internal and external sphincters of the urethra.

Furthermore, the pelvic floor muscles have an important role in maintaining the continence mechanism and pelvic organ support [3], thereby indicating that strengthening the pelvic floor muscles may help prevent urine leakage with increased intra-abdominal pressure.

Pregnancy is one of the main risk factors for the development of UI in young women [4, 5] because pregnancy may be associated with reduced strength of the pelvic floor muscles which can develop into UI. Interestingly, most women (76%) perceive that they have UI due to weakened pelvic floor muscles [6]. Studies in pregnant women with SUI have found significantly decreased pelvic floor muscle strength in incontinent pregnant women as compared with continent pregnant women [7, 8].

Pregnancy may be associated with reduced pelvic floor muscle strength which can develop into SUI. However, the exact causes of pregnancy-related SUI remain unclear [9, 10]. Both physiological and hormonal changes during pregnancy may lead to disruption of normal urinary tract function and reduced strength of the supportive and sphincteric function of the pelvic floor muscles. Hence, when intra-abdominal pressure increases, the urethral sphincter is not strong enough to close the urethra. The result is urine leakage [11].

Urinary incontinence is common in women and can have a substantial impact on individual quality of life (QoL) [12]. Although UI is not a life-threatening disorder, it deeply affects a woman's QoL [13]. It is a condition that causes considerable distress in the form of physical discomfort, economic burden, shame and loss of self-confidence, not to mention sexual function, thereby diminishing quality of life [14, 15].

Therefore, UI can affect the psychological and social well-being of women with long-term effects on QoL and is associated with enormous health-related costs. Urinary incontinence is also known to have detrimental effects on QoL in approximately 54.3% of all pregnant women [16]. Pregnant women with UI have statistically significant lower QoL during pregnancy than those without UI [17], and the QoL of incontinent pregnant women worsens with increasing gestational age until term [18]. Pregnant women with UUI or MUI have worse QoL scores during pregnancy than those with SUI alone [19].

Urinary incontinence not only affects QoL during pregnancy, but also affects QoL during postpartum period. Therefore, UI is a serious health problem during the postpartum period and affects the QoL of postpartum women by disrupting daily activities [20]. Postpartum women who have UI are associated with feelings of frustration and embarrassment, in addition, the women report that UI diminished their ability to have sexual relations and reduced involvement in physical and recreational activities [21]. Mascarenhas et al. [17] found women with UI during pregnancy and childbirth have a worse QoL than continent women. Furthermore, the prevalence of depressive symptoms is also higher in women with UI that those without UI. Women who have urinary incontinence after delivery are more likely to develop postpartum depression than those without urinary incontinence [22]. In cross-sectional study, Hullfish et al. [23] found that UUI was associated with postpartum depression at 6 weeks after delivery. Interestingly, postpartum UI not only develops postpartum depression, but also develops anxiety after delivery. In prospective cohort study, Goyeneche et al. [24] also found that QoL was associated with anxiety in the postpartum period. Moreover, women who have UI during pregnancy or postpartum period have significant risk factors for increasing UI later in life [25].

In this chapter, the researcher will present data from several studies of UI in pregnant and postpartum women for the purpose of reviewing and discussing the prevalence, types and severity of UI among women from pregnancy to the postpartum period. Understanding these issues can be useful for healthcare professionals in delivering more informed counseling for women to help prevent UI during pregnancy and the postpartum period.

PREVALENCE AND TYPES OF URINARY INCONTINENCE MOST COMMONLY ENCOUNTERED IN WOMEN DURING PREGNANCY

A number of studies have been conducted on the prevalence of UI during pregnancy. The range of UI prevalence varies with the prevalence of UI in the population depending on the use of different study designs, definitions, evaluations, questionnaires and stage of pregnancy in which data were collected [25-27]. Although most population data have focused on European or Western countries, a few studies have discovered UI during pregnancy in Asia, especially in South East Asia.

Many studies in European, Western, Asian and South East Asian countries have investigated the prevalence of UI in antepartum and postpartum women with different populations, objectives and methodology. In Denmark, Viktrup et al. [28] researchers found 4% of primiparous women to have had SUI before pregnancy and 32% during pregnancy, whereas 7% developed postpartum SUI. In Germany, Huebner et al. [29] reported data from primigravidous women that UI was estimated at 26.3% and significantly increased during the second half of pregnancy. In Spain, Diez-Itza et al. [30] conducted an observational study to investigate the incidence and severity of SUI in 458 primigravidous women at term and its association with maternal body weight. They reported the prevalence of SUI among 596 primigravidous women to be 30.3%. In another cross-sectional study from Spain, Martínez Franco et al. [31] conducted a study to determine the prevalence and severity of UI between the first and third trimesters of pregnancy. They found the incidence of UI during pregnancy to be different in the first and third trimesters (18.96% and 39.76%, respectively). They also found all (100%) and most women (84.12%) with UI during the first and third trimesters, respectively, to leak urine in small amounts. Those women mainly presented with SUI (78.37%) and UUI was only present in 12.16%. Therefore, the prevalence of UI was found to be 34.37%, which means that this disorder is more common during the third trimester of pregnancy than the first.

In a cohort study from Spain, Solans-Domènech et al. [32] conducted a study to estimate frequency and severity in addition to identifying the risk factors of UI and anal incontinence (AI) during pregnancy and after delivery in previously continent nulliparous women. During pregnancy, the researchers found the cumulative incidence rate of UI to be 39.1% (95% CI 36.3-41.9) with a rate of 10.3% (95% CI 8.3-12.3) for AI.

In Norway, Morkved and Bø [33] conducted a study to investigate the prevalence of SUI during pregnancy and the postpartum period. According to the findings, the prevalence of UI during pregnancy was 42%; at 8 weeks after delivery, the prevalence of self-reported UI was 38%. It can be concluded, therefore, that the prevalence of UI is nearly the same at 8 weeks postpartum as during pregnancy. In another study from Norway, Wesnes et al. [34] participated in the Norwegian Mother and Child Cohort Study at the Norwegian Institute of Public Health to investigate the incidence and prevalence of UI during pregnancy and associated risk factors in 43,279 pregnant women. In the third trimester, SUI was reported to be the most common type of UI during pregnancy experienced by 31% of nulliparous and 42% of multiparous women.

In the *United Kingdom,* Mason et al. [35] found 59% of pregnant women to report SUI during pregnancy; 10% of these women had daily episodes of incontinence during pregnancy. In another prospective study from the *United Kingdom,* Elenskaia et al. [36] evaluated changes in pelvic organ support, pelvic floor symptoms and their effect on QoL during the first pregnancy in nulliparous women. According to the findings, the symptoms and discomfort with voiding difficulties and SUI increased from the second to the third trimesters of pregnancy. In a cross-sectional survey from North-East Scotland, Whitford et al. [37] conducted a study to establish the prevalence of SUI in women during the third trimester of pregnancy. According to the findings, the prevalence of SUI in pregnant women was 54.3%.

In Australia, Chiarelli and Campbell [38] found 64% of 304 women to report incontinence during pregnancy. Similar to this finding in a cohort study from Australia, Brown et al. [39] found the prevalence of UI to increase from 10.8% in the 12 months before the index pregnancy to 55.9% during the third trimester. Stress urinary incontinence (36.9%) and MUI (13.1%) were more common during pregnancy than UUI alone (5.9%).

The prevalence of UI in Asia is lower compared with Europe. In a large population survey conducted in China among 10,098 Chinese primiparous women, SUI was estimated to be present in 18.6% of pregnant women in late pregnancy [40]. One the prevalence of SUI in Taiwanese primiparous women, 26.7% of the women reported SUI [41]. In another survey, the prevalence of SUI in pregnant women was reported to be 46.1% [42]. In South Asia, a survey was conducted in India in which the prevalence of SUI was found to be 19.2% [43]. In South East Asia, the prevalence of UI during pregnancy has been found to be approximately 36.5% [44] in Thailand. In another study from Malaysia, Abdullah et al. [45] investigated the prevalence of UI among primigravida during the third trimester. The findings on the prevalence of UI during the third trimester was 34.3% with stress incontinence (64.8%) as the most commonly encountered, followed by MUI (24.8%) and UUI (6.7%). A study from the Middle East conducted in Jordan reported the estimated SUI to be approximately 45% of pregnant women [46]. In another cross-sectional study from Turkey, Erbil et al. [47] conducted a study to investigate effects on QoL and determine the frequency and risk factors for UI among 502 pregnant Turkish women. According to the findings, %40.4of pregnant women reported UI. Approximately, three-fourths (%78.8) of pregnant women with UI had SUI in which %14.8had mixed UI and %6.4had UUI.

In North America, the highest reported prevalence of SUI is in the United States. According to data from the US, Thomason et al. [48] reported a prevalence of 60% for SUI during pregnancy in continent primiparous women. In another study, Raza-Khan et al. [49] reported UI in 70% of nulliparous and 75% of multiparous women with 32% reporting pure SUI. In South America, Brazil, Oliveira et al. [50] investigated the prevalence of UI and the risk factors correlated with UI in relation to socio-demographic variables and QoL. Based on the findings, 71% of the subjects had UI during the last four weeks of pregnancy. It can be concluded, therefore, that the majority of pregnant women have UI that negatively affects their QoL. In another study from Brazil, the prevalence of SUI in healthy pregnant Brazilian women was reported to be 46.1% in primigravidous women and 54.0% in multigravidous women [51].

In West Africa, a cross-sectional study was conducted in Zaria, Nigeria, by Adaji et al. [52] to establish the prevalence of lower urinary symptoms of discomfort during pregnancy among 204 pregnant women. According to the findings, the prevalence of SUI during the second trimester of pregnancy was 12.9% with a rate of 12.9% for UUI. During the third trimester, the women also reported the prevalence of SUI and UUI to be 16.1% and 7.5%, respectively.

In a multi-ethnic population, Bø et al. [53] investigated the prevalence of UI in a multi-ethnic population of pregnant women. The prevalence rates for UI at 28 weeks of gestation were 26% for women of African origin, 36% for women of Middle Eastern origin, 40% for women of East Asian origin, 43% for women of South Asian origin and 45% for women of European/North American origin. The differences were significant between women of African and European/North American origins and between women of African and South Asian origins. Age and parity were also found to be positively associated with the prevalence of UI during pregnancy. A descriptive correlational study that was similar to the study of Spellacy et al. [54] described the incidence of UI during pregnancy and the puerperium period to identify potential contributing factors. According to the findings, the racial distribution of those reporting UI was as follows: Caucasian (70%; 21 out of 30); African American (44%; 8 out of 18) and Hispanic/Asian (100%; n = 2). Of the women who reported UI during the first interview, 7 women (50%) continued to experience UI from 4 to 6 weeks postpartum. Of the participants experiencing postpartum UI, 77% (n = 7) were Caucasians.

In a multicenter prospective pregnancy cohort study, Brown et al. [39] reported the prevalence of SUI to be 36.9%, further reporting that SUI was more common during pregnancy than urge incontinence in nulliparous women.

Although the prevalence of UI various worldwide, numerous studies have shown the prevalence rates for SUI between 13% and 19% during the first trimester of pregnancy [55, 56] to increase during the second trimester and peak during the third trimester to rates of 19.2% and 37.5%, respectively [41]. Most studies have found the prevalence of SUI to generally increase with gestational age [41, 42, 57], peaking during the third trimester, followed by the second and first trimesters [58, 59]. According to the study of Van Kerrebroeck et al. [60], the prevalence of incontinence worsens as pregnancy advances and a rate of 17-25% is reported for UI in pregnant women during early pregnancy with an increase to 36-37% in late pregnancy. Similar findings were reported by Wijma et al. [59] who found the high prevalence of UI during pregnancy to be 30% for women at gestational ages of 28-32 weeks and 35% for pregnant women at gestational ages of 36-38 weeks

According to the above findings in this summary, the prevalence of UI during pregnancy was found to vary depending on the use of different populations, study designs, methods of assessing incontinence, definitions of UI, evaluation questionnaire and stage of pregnancy. Therefore, the prevalence of UI during pregnancy has been estimated to range from 10.8% to 84.12%. The prevalence of UI was also found to increase with gestational age and peak during the third trimester of pregnancy. SUI is the most common type of UI during pregnancy with an overall prevalence rate ranged from 4.0% to 78.8% with greater prevalence than MUI (13.1% to 24.8%) and UUI (5.9% to 12.9%).

PREVALENCE AND TYPES OF URINARY INCONTINENCE MOST COMMONLY ENCOUNTERED IN WOMEN DURING THE POSTPARTUM PERIOD

Mason et al. [35] conducted a study to examine the prevalence of SUI during and after pregnancy in 1,008 women. According to the findings, the prevalence of SUI was 59% during pregnancy and 31% following delivery. In a prospective, longitudinal study, Chaliha et al. [61] investigated the effects of pregnancy and delivery on continence to assess whether the physical markers of collagen weakness can predict postpartum urinary and fecal incontinence in 549 nulliparous women. The prevalence of UI before, during, and after pregnancy was also found to be 3.6%, 43.7% and 14.6%, while the rates of fecal incontinence were 0.7%, 6.0% and 5.5%, respectively. Fecal urgency has been found to be more common in women with spontaneous and instrument-assisted vaginal deliveries (n = 413) compared to cesarean deliveries (n = 131) (7.3% versus 3.1%; P = .046).

In another survey from China, Zhu et al. [40] conducted a study to characterize the risk factors of UI during late pregnancy and the postpartum period in 10,098 primiparous women. After delivery, the women with no UI in late pregnancy were found to have a prevalence of newly developed UI cases at rates of 3.7% and 3.0% at 6 weeks and 6 months postpartum, respectively. The prevalence of all UI was also found to be 26.7% in late pregnancy, 9.5% at 6 weeks postpartum and 6.8% at 6 months postpartum. Furthermore, most cases involved SUI (18.6%, 6.9% and 5.0% in late pregnancy, and at 6 weeks and 6 months postpartum, respectively). Martin-Martin et al. [62] conducted a prospective study to determine the prevalence of UI before pregnancy, in the third trimester and at 3 and 6 months postpartum in 413 pregnant women. According to the findings, the prevalence of UI during the third trimester was 31%. During the postpartum period, the prevalence of UI was found to be 11.3% at 3 months and 6.9% at 6 months postpartum. It can be concluded, therefore, that the prevalence of UI after delivery was higher in women with UI during pregnancy and lower in cases caesarean sections. Tanawattanacharoen and Thongtawee [63] conducted a study to assess the prevalence of UI during the late third trimester and three months postpartum period. Based on the findings, the prevalence of UI during late pregnancy and at three months postpartum were 53.8% and 7.8%, respectively. This difference reached statistical significance (p < 0.001). There were 53.5% of SUI, 20% of UUI and 7.8% of MUI late during the third trimester, whereas only SUI was found at three months postpartum. It can be concluded, therefore, that the prevalence of UI is quite high late during the third trimester (53.8%) and decreased significantly at three months postpartum (7.8%).

The prospective study of Eftekhar et al. [64], was aimed at assessing the prevalence of postpartum SUI, the relationship between postpartum SUI and mode of delivery; and the association between SUI and other obstetric factors in 1,000 primiparous women with no history of UI. According to the findings, the prevalence of postpartum SUI was 14.1%, and the mode of delivery was significantly associated with SUI. The prevalence rates were 15.9% after vaginal delivery, 10.7% after elective cesarean section (CS) and 25% after CS performed for obstructed labor. In a cross-sectional epidemiological study, Lopes et al. [65] attempted to affirm the prevalence of self-reported UI in women after childbirth in 288 women. Based on the findings, the prevalence of self-reported postpartum UI was .%24.6

Hvidman et al. [66] conducted a questionnaire-based cross-sectional survey to identify the pre-pregnancy, pregnancy and delivery correlates of postpartum UI. According to findings, the prevalence rates for UI immediately after childbirth and at 6 months postpartum were reported at 23.4% and 2.7%, respectively. Similarly, Lewicky-Gaupp et al. [67] conducted a study to determine the prevalence of urinary and anal incontinence during pregnancy and the immediate postpartum period. During the third trimester, 44% of patients complained of urinary urge incontinence and 43% complained of stress incontinence, while 12% of the subjects complained of fecal and 41% of flatal incontinence, only 9% complained of UUI and 5% of SUI at 6 weeks postpartum. Burgio et al. [68] conducted a study to describe the prevalence and severity of UI during the 12-month postpartum period in 523 women. At 6 weeks postpartum, 11.36% of the women reported some degree of UI since the index delivery.

Another survey by Pregazzi et al. [69] was conducted to assess the prevalence of urinary symptoms at 3 months after vaginal delivery, the relationship between urinary symptoms and vaginal descent, and the association between urinary symptoms and obstetric factors in 537 women. After 3 months postpartum, the prevalence of SUI was reported to be 8.2% in primiparous women and 20% in multiparous women. Urge incontinence was present in 5.5% of primiparous women and in 13% of multiparous women.

Therefore, it can be concluded that UI appears to be associated with induced labor with prostaglandins and general maternal factors such as parity and elevated weight in early pregnancy. Wilson et al. [70] conducted a study to examine the correlations between obstetric factors and the prevalence of UI at 3 months after delivery. At three months postpartum, 34.3% of the women admitted to some degree of UI with 3.3% having daily or more frequent leakage. In a population-based survey, Boyles et al. [71] conducted a study to estimate the effects of the mode of delivery on the incidence of UI at 3-6 months postpartum in 15,787 primiparous women. According to the findings, a total of 955 women (17.1%) reported leakage of urine. No statistical differences were found in the incidence of UI among women who had elective cesarean deliveries (6.1%), women who had cesarean deliveries after labor (5.7%) and women who had cesarean deliveries after labor and pushing (6.4%). It can be concluded, therefore, that UI is common during the immediate postpartum period after a woman's first pregnancy.

Baydock et al. [72] conducted a study to determine the prevalence of and risk factors for urinary and fecal incontinence at 4 months after vaginal delivery in women who had had vaginal deliveries. According to the findings, 145 women (23%) had SUI, 77 women (12%) had UUI, 181 women (29%) had UI and 23 women (4%) had fecal incontinence. It can be concluded, therefore, that UI is common in women at 4 months postpartum and fecal incontinence is less common in women during the postpartum period. In a prospective pregnancy cohort study, Gartland et al. [73] investigated the contribution of obstetric risk factors and the prevalence of persistent UI between 4 and 18 months postpartum in 1,507 nulliparous women. Of the women who were continent before pregnancy, the prevalence of UI at 4 and 18 months postpartum was reported at 44% and 25%, respectively. Compared with spontaneous vaginal births, women who had had a caesarean section before labor (aOR 0.4, 95% CI 0.2–0.9), in first stage of labor (aOR 0.4, 95% CI 0.2–0.6) or in second stage of labor (aOR 0.4, 95% CI 0.2–1.0) were less likely to report persistent UI at 4–18 months postpartum. Prolonged second-stage labor in women who had an operative vaginal birth was associated with increased likelihood of UI (aOR 2.5, 95% CI 1.3–4.6). Compared with women who were continent in pregnancy, women reporting UI in pregnancy had a seven-fold increase in the likelihood of persistent UI (aOR 7.4, 95% CI 5.1–10.7). Therefore, it can be concluded that persistent UI is common after childbirth and more likely following prolonged labor in combination with operative vaginal birth. The majority of women reporting persistent UI at 4–18 months postpartum also experienced symptoms during pregnancy.

In a longitudinal cohort study (EDEN cohort), Quiboeuf et al. [74] conducted a cohort study to describe the risk factors associated with the prevalence, incidence and remission of UI between 4 and 24 months postpartum. According to the findings, the prevalence of postpartum UI is 20.7% at 4 months and 19.9% at 24 months. Furthermore, the likelihood of UI remission at 24 months is 51.9% and caesarean delivery has been found to be associated with increased likelihood of UI remission [0.43 (0.19-0.97)].

Wesnes et al. [75] conducted a cohort study to investigate the prevalence of UI at 6 months postpartum in 12,679 primigravidous women who were continent before pregnancy. According to the findings, the prevalence of UI was reported by 31% of women at 6 months after delivery. Compared with women who were continent during pregnancy, incontinence was more prevalent at 6 months after delivery among women who had experienced incontinence during pregnancy (adjusted RR 2.3, 95% CI 2.2-2.4). It can be concluded, therefore, that UI is prevalent at 6 months postpartum. Hatem et al. [76] conducted a study to identify the factors associated with UI, anal AI and combined UI and AI (UI/AI) in 2,492 primiparous women in Quebec at six months postpartum. According to the findings, the prevalence was 29.6% for UI, 20.6% for AI and 10.4% for combined UI/AI.

In a prospective cohort study, Hansen et al. [77] investigated the impact of first pregnancy and delivery on the prevalence and types of UI during pregnancy and at 1 year after delivery in nulliparous and primiparous women. During pregnancy, the prevalence of any type of UI in the primiparous group was found to be 32.1%, compared to 13.8% in the nulliparous group (Adjusted OR = 3.3; 95%CI = 2.4-4.4). At one year after delivery, the prevalence in the primiparous group was also found to be 29.3% compared to 16.6% in the nulliparous group (Adjusted OR = 2.5; 95%CI =1.8-3.5). It can be concluded, therefore, that the prevalence of UI during pregnancy is 3.3 times higher in comparison with nulliparous women. After 1 year, the difference was reduced, but still 2.5 times higher in the primiparous group.

In a prospective longitudinal study, Chang et al. [78] examined the association between vaginal or cesarean delivery and UI and identified the trend for changes in UI within the first 12 months postpartum. Based on the findings, the vaginal delivery group had significantly higher prevalence of UI at 4-6 weeks and at 3, 6 and 12 months (29.1-40.2% vaginal compared with 14.2-25.5% cesarean deliveries); SUI at 4-6 weeks and 3 and 12 months (15.9-25.4% vaginal compared with 6.4-15.6% cesarean deliveries); and moderate or severe UI at 3-5 days, 4-6 weeks and 6 months (7.9-18.5% vaginal compared with 4.3-11.3% cesarean deliveries); and a significant higher score for interference in daily life at 3-5 days and 4-6 weeks (1.0, 0.7 vaginal compared with 0.7, 0.4 cesarean) compared with those in the cesarean delivery group.

In a longitudinal study, Diez-Itza et al. [79] investigated the risk factors involved in SUI at 1 year after first delivery in 352 primigravidous women. According to the findings, SUI affected 40 (11.4%) women at 1 year after first delivery with an incontinence severity index (ISI) distribution of 62.5% slight, 32.5% moderate, 2.5% severe and 2.5% very severe SUI. According to the findings, new onset of SUI during pregnancy is an independent risk factor for SUI during the postpartum period. Schytt, et al. [25] conducted a cohort study to describe the prevalence of SUI at 1year after childbirth in 2,390 national samples of Swedish-speaking women. At one year after birth, 22%of the women were found to have symptoms of SUI. It can be concluded, therefore, that SUI at 1year after childbirth is a common symptom that could possibly be reduced by identifying women with urinary leakage at postnatal check-ups. In a cohort study, Brown et al. [80] found the prevalence to be 47% for UI and 17% for fecal incontinence during the first 12 months postpartum.

In another cross-sectional study, Ege et al. [20] attempted to determine the prevalence of UI during the 12-month postpartum period and the risk factors related to this condition in 1,749 postpartum women. According to the findings, 12.7% of the women had suffered from UI prior to pregnancy, 42.0% had experienced UI during pregnancy and 19.5% had complained of the condition during the postpartum period. At 12 months after childbirth, 19.5% of the women reported experiencing varying degrees of urinary incontinence. While 42.2% of the women suffered from SUI, 10.3% had UUI, 47.5% complained of a MUI, 7.3% reported leakage of urine during sexual intercourse and 14.4% reported the need to use protective pads. According to the findings, 12.3% of the women performed pelvic floor muscle exercises and only 15.2% had consulted their doctors about UI. Chan et al. [81] conducted a study to evaluate the factors and prevalence associated with UI and FI during and after a woman's first pregnancy in nulliparous Chinese women. According to the findings, the prevalence of antenatal UI increased with gestation. Twelve months after delivery, the women also reported the prevalence of SUI, UUI and FI to be 25.9% (95% CI 21.5–30.6), 8.2% (95% CI 5.2–11.2) and 4.0% (95% CI 1.9–6.1), respectively,

In another cross-sectional study, Barbosal et al. [82] assessed the two-year postpartum prevalence of UI and pelvic floor muscle dysfunction and the causal factors of UI in 220 women. At 2 years after delivery, the findings indicated the prevalence of UI to be 17% following vaginal childbirth and

18.9% following cesarean section. The only risk factor for pelvic floor muscle dysfunction was weight gain during pregnancy.

Herrmann et al. [83] conducted a longitudinal cohort study to estimate the incidence of postpartum SUI at 3 years after delivery and its correlation with mode of delivery and parity in 120 women. The findings indicated a significant difference in the incidence of postpartum SUI among patients with SUI during pregnancy (p > 0.0001). Women that were asymptomatic during pregnancy and had vaginal deliveries developed SUI 2.4 times more frequently than women who had c-sections (19.2% and 8.0%, respectively). The incidence of SUI after delivery dropped significantly in primiparous women (p = 0.0073) and multiparous women with two or three deliveries (p < 0.0001), but not in multiparous women with four or more deliveries (66.7% to 60.0%) (p = 0.5637).

In a prospective pregnancy cohort study, Gartland et al. [84] investigated the frequency, severity and risk factors for urinary and fecal incontinence at 4 years after a first birth in 1,011 nulliparous women. At 4 years postpartum, 29.6% of the women reported UI and 7.1% reported fecal incontinence. The women who reported UI before or during the index pregnancy and those experiencing symptoms during the first year postpartum had increased odds for incontinence at 4 years. Based on their findings, urinary and fecal incontinence are prevalent conditions at 4 years after a first birth. Women reporting urinary or fecal incontinence during pregnancy are markedly more likely to report symptoms at 4 years postpartum. At 4 years after first delivery, Fritel et al. [85] found the prevalence of UI to be 22%, the prevalence of AI to be 6.5%, and the prevalence of UI and AI to be 6.5%.

Liang et al. [86] conducted a study to investigate the prevalence and contributing factors of UI in primiparous women at 5 years after their first birth and to evaluate the associations of UI with delivery mode and quality of life. At five years after first delivery, the prevalence of SUI and UUI were found to be 43.6 % and 19.2%, respectively. The findings also indicated that women with UI during their first pregnancy were more likely to develop UI 5 years postpartum than those without UI; women who delivered their first child vaginally had a greater incidence of UI than those having cesarean births; UUI in women following cesarean delivery has more negative effects on emotional health than UUI following vaginal birth, whereas the impact of SUI does not significantly differ between delivery groups. Therefore, it can be concluded that UI during the first pregnancy and vaginal delivery in primiparous women may predict an increased risk for UI 5 years after delivery. UUI adversely affects women's emotional health, especially in women who have had cesarean sections.

In a longitudinal study, MacArthur et al. [87] investigated the prevalence of persistent UI (at three months and six years after the index birth) and long-term postpartum UI (at six years after the index birth) in addition to correlations with the mode of first and subsequent deliveries. The prevalence of persistent UI was found to be 24%.

In a longitudinal cohort study, Viktrup et al. [88] estimated the impact of SUI onset in first pregnancy or the postpartum period as well as the risk for symptoms 12 years after the first delivery in 241 women. Twelve years after first delivery, the prevalence of SUI was found to be 42% with an incidence rate of 30%. Moreover, the prevalence of SUI at 12 years after first pregnancy and delivery was found to be significantly higher (P < .01) in women with onset during first pregnancy (56%, 37 of 66) and in women with onset shortly after delivery (78%, 14 of 18) compared to those without initial symptoms (30% at 44 of 146). In 70 women who had onset of symptoms during first pregnancy or shortly after the delivery, but remission at 3 months postpartum, a total of 40 (57%) had SUI 12 years later. In 11 women with onset of symptoms during the first pregnancy or shortly after delivery, but no remission at 3 months postpartum, a total of 10 (91%) had SUI 12 years later. It can be concluded, therefore, that the onset of SUI during first pregnancy or the puerperal period carries an increased the risk for long-lasting symptoms.

In a twelve-year longitudinal cohort study, MacArthur et al. [89] investigated the extent of persistent UI 12 years after birth and association with delivery-mode history as well as other factors. According to the findings, the prevalence of persistent UI at 12 years after childbirth was 37.9%. Among those who had reported UI at 3 months, 76.4% also reported UI at 12 years.

In a registry-based national cohort study, Gyhagen et al. [90] investigated the prevalence and risk factors for symptomatic pelvic organ prolapse (sPOP) and sPOP concomitant factors with UI in 5,236 women at 20 years after one vaginal or caesarean delivery. Based on the findings, the prevalence of sPOP was higher after vaginal delivery than after caesarean section (14.6 versus 6.3%, [OR 2.55; 95% CI 1.98–3.28]).

According to the above findings in this summary, the number of postpartum women with UI is variable. Therefore, the prevalence of UI during the postpartum period ranges from 2.7% to 76.4%. SUI is the most common type of UI which found at rates from 5.0% to 57% in women following delivery.

As previously mentioned, it can be concluded that UI is a common disorder among postpartum women. Furthermore, many risk factors contribute to the development of UI such as UI before pregnancy, UI during pregnancy, increased weight gain during pregnancy, parity and mode of delivery. The pathogenesis of postpartum UI includes not only the effects of pelvic floor trauma on urethrovesical mobility under stress, but also a deficiency in urethral resistance caused by drugs such as prostaglandins.

The prevalence of UI in postpartum women is encountered from immediately after delivery to 6 weeks postpartum within a short-term period from 3 to 6 months postpartum, within a long-term period from 1 to 6 years and at 12 and 20 years after delivery. The present study concludes that types of incontinence are classified into the following 6 groups: UI, SUI, UUI, MUI, FI and leak incontinence.

According to the findings, the highest prevalence of UI was reported at 76.4% among postpartum women during 12 years after delivery. The lowest prevalence rate of UI at 6 months postpartum was 2.7%. For any types of UI during the postpartum period, SUI was found to be the most common type of UI in postpartum women. The highest prevalence of SUI was reported at 57.0% among postpartum women during the first 12 years after delivery. The lowest prevalence rate of SUI at 6 months postpartum was 5%, followed by the highest prevalence of UUI that was reported at 44% among postpartum women during the postpartum period. The lowest prevalence rate of UUI at 3 months of the postpartum period was 5.5%. The highest prevalence of MUI was reported at 47.5% among postpartum women during the first 12 months of the postpartum period.

In this summary, the prevalence of UI during the postpartum period was found to vary, depending on the use of different populations, study designs, methods of assessing incontinence, definitions of UI, evaluation questionnaires and time elapsed since childbirth. Therefore, it can be concluded that the prevalence of UI peaks during pregnancy and decreases after childbirth. During the postpartum period, the overall prevalence of postpartum UI ranges from 2.7% to 76.4% with a remission rate at three months after childbirth of up to 86.4%. The most common type of UI in postpartum women is SUI in which the prevalence ranges from 5.0% to 57.0%, followed by MUI (47.5%), UUI (5.5% to 44.0%). The prevalence of fecal incontinence ranges from 4.0% to 12.0%.

REFERENCES

[1]   Haylen, B. T., de Ridder, D., Freeman, R. M., et al. (2010). An International Urogynecological Association (IUGA)/International Continence Society (ICS) joint report on the terminology for female pelvic floor dysfunction. *Int Urogynecol J*, *21*(1), 5–26.

[2]   Long, R. M., Giri, S. K. and Flood, H. D. (2008). Current concepts in female stress urinary incontinence. *Surgeon*, *6*(6), 366-372.

[3]   Handa, V. L., Harris, T. A. and Ostergard, D. R. (1996). Protecting the pelvic floor: obstetric management to prevent incontinence and pelvic organ prolapse. *Obstet Gynecol*, *88*, 470-478.

[4]   Morkved, S. and Bo, K. (2000). Effect of postpartum pelvic floor muscle training in prevention and treatment of urinary incontinence: a one-year follow up. *Br J Obstet Gynaecol*, *107*(8), 1022-1028.

[5]   Peyrat, L., Haillot, O., Bruyere, F., Boutin, J. M., Bertrand, P. and Lanson, Y. (2002). Prevalence and risk factors of urinary incontinence in young and middle-aged women. *BJU Int*, *89*, 61-66.

[6]   Hermansen, I. L., O'Connell, B. and Gaskin, C. J. (2010). Are postpartum women in denmark being given helpful information about urinary incontinence and pelvic floor exercises? *J Midwifery Womens Health*, *55*(2), 171-174.

[7]   Hilde, G., Stær-Jensen, J., Ellström Engh, M., Brækken, I. H. and Bø, K. (2012). Continence and pelvic floor status in nulliparous women at midterm pregnancy. *Int Urogynecol J*, *23*(9), 1257-1263.

[8]   Morkved, S., Salvesen, K. A., Bo, K. and Eik-Nes, S. (2004). Pelvic floor muscle strength and thickness in continent and incontinent nulliparous pregnant women. *Int Urogynecol J Pelvic Floor Dysfunct*, *15*, 384-390.

[9]   Mikhail, M. S. and Anyaegbunam, A. (1995). Lower Urinary Tract Dysfunction in pregnancy: a review. *Obstet Gynecol Surv*, *50*(9), 675-683.

[10] Viktrup, L. (2002). The risk of urinary tract symptom five years after the first delivery. *Neurourol Urodyn*, *21*(1), 2-29.

[11] Sangsawang, B. and Sangsawang, N. (2013). Stress urinary incontinence in pregnant women: a review of prevalence, pathophysiology, and treatment. *Int Urogynecol J*, *24*, 901–12.

[12] Kocaöz, S., Talas, M. S. and Atabekoğlu, C. S. (2010). Urinary incontinence in pregnant women and their quality of life. *J Clin Nurs*, *19*(23-24), 3314-3323.

[13] Cerruto, M. A., D'Elia, C., Aloisi, A., Fabrello, M. and Artibani, W. (2013). Prevalence, incidence and obstetric factors' impact on female urinary incontinence in Europe: a systematic review. *Urol Int, 90*(1), 1-9.

[14] Norton, P. A. (1990). Prevalence and social impact of urinary incontinence in women. *Clin Obstet Gynecol, 33*(2), 295-297.

[15] Temml, C., Haidinger, G., Schmidbauer, J., Schatzl, G. and Madersbacher, S. (2000). Urinary incontinence in both sexes: prevalence rates and impact on quality of life and sexual life. *Neurourol Urodyn., 19*(3), 259-271.

[16] Dolan, L. M., Walsh, D., Hamilton, S., Marshall, K., Thompson, K. and Ashe, R. G. (2004). A study of quality of life in primigravidae with urinary incontinence. *Int Urogynecol J Pelvic Floor Dysfunct, 15*, 160–164.

[17] Mascarenhas, T., Coelho, R., Oliveira, M. and Patricio, B. (2003). Impact of urinary incontinence on quality of life during pregnancy and after childbirth. Paper presented at the 33rd annual meeting of the International Continence Society, Florence, Italy, 5th - 9th October, 2003.

[18] van de Pol, G. G., Van Brummen, H. J., Bruinse, H. W., Heintz, A. P. and van der Vaart, C. H. (2007). Is there an association between depressive and urinary symptoms during and after pregnancy? *Int Urogynecol J Pelvic Floor Dysfunct, 18*, 1409–1415.

[19] van Brummen, H. J., Bruinse, H. W., Van de Pol, G., Heintz, A. P. and Van der Vaart, C. H. (2006). What is the effect of overactive bladder symptoms on woman's quality of life during and after first pregnancy? *BJU Int, 97*(2), 296–300.

[20] Ege, E., Akin, B., Altuntug, K., Benli, S. and Arioz, A. (2008). Prevalence of urinary incontinence in the 12-month postpartum period and related risk factors in Turkey. *Urol Int, 80*(4), 355-61.

[21] Hermansen, I. L., O'Connell, B. O. and Gaskin, C. J. (2010). Women's explanations for urinary incontinence, their management strategies, and their quality of life during the postpartum period. *Wound Ostomy Continence Nurs, 37*(2), 187-92.

[22] Sword, W., Landy, C. K., Thabane, L., et al. (2011). Is mode of delivery associated with postpartum depression at 6 weeks: a prospective cohort study. *Br J Obstet Gynaecol, 118*(8), 966-77.

[23] Hullfish, K. L., Fenner, D. E., Sorser, S. A., Visger, J., Clayton, A. and Steers, W. D. (2007). Postpartum Depression, Urge Urinary

Incontinence, and Overactive Bladder Syndrome: Is There an Association? *Int Urogynecol J Pelvic Floor Dysfunct, 18*(10), 1121-6.

[24] Goyeneche, L., Uranga, S., Salgueiro, M. D., Lekuona, A., Sarasqueta, C. and Diez Itza, I. (2013). Influence of urinary incontinence on postpartum depression and anxiety. Paper presented at the 43rd annual meeting of the International Continence Society, Barcelona, Spain, 26th - 30th August, 2013.

[25] Schytt, E., Lindmark, G. and Waldenstrom, U. (2004) Symptoms of stress incontinence 1 year after childbirth: prevalence and predictors in a national Swedish sample. *Acta Obstet Gynecol Scand, 83*, 928–936.

[26] Viktrup, L. and Lose, G. (2001). The risk of stress incontinence 5 after first delivery. *Am J Obstet Gynecol, 185*(1), 82-87.

[27] Thom, D. H. and Rortveit, G. (2010). Prevalence of postpartum urinary incontinence: a systematic review. *Acta Obstet Gynecol Scand, 89*(12), 1511-1522.

[28] Viktrup, L., Lose, G., Rolff, M. and Barford, K. (1992). The symptom of stress incontinence caused by pregnancy or delivery in primiparas. *Obstet Gynecol, 79*, 945-949.

[29] Huebner, M., Antolic, A. and Tunn, R. (2010). The impact of pregnancy and vaginal delivery on urinary incontinence. *Int J Gynecol Obstet, 110*(3), 249-251.

[30] Diez-Itza, I., Ibañez, L., Arrue, M., Paredes, J., Murgiondo, A. and Sarasqueta, C. (2009). Influence of maternal weight on the new onset of stress urinary incontinence in pregnant women. *Int Urogynecol J Pelvic Floor Dysfunct, 20*(10), 1259-1263.

[31] Martínez Franco, E., Parés, D., Lorente Colomé, N., Méndez Paredes, J. R. and Amat Tardiu, L. (2014). Urinary incontinence during pregnancy. Is there a difference between first and third trimester? *Eur J Obstet Gynecol Reprod Biol, 182*, 86-90.

[32] Solans-Domènech, M., Sánchez, E., Espuña-Pons, M. and Pelvic Floor Research Group (Grup de Recerca del Sòl Pelvià; GRESP). (2010). Urinary and anal incontinence during pregnancy and postpartum: incidence, severity, and risk factors. *Obstet Gynecol, 115*(3), 618-28.

[33] Mørkved, S. and Bø, K. (1999). Prevalence of urinary incontinence during pregnancy and postpartum. *Int Urogynecol J Pelvic Floor Dysfunct, 10*, 394-398.

[34] Wesnes, S. L., Rortveit, G., Bø, K. and Hunskaar, S. (2007). Urinary incontinence during pregnancy. *Obstet Gynecol, 109*(4), 922-928.

[35] Mason, L., Glenn, S., Walton, I. and Appletion, C. (1999). The prevalence of stress incontinence during pregnancy and following delivery. *Midwifery, 15*(2), 120-128.

[36] Elenskaia, K., Thakar, R., Sultan, A. H., Scheer, I. and Onwude, J. (2013). Pelvic organ support, symptoms and quality of life during pregnancy: a prospective study. *Int Urogynecol J, 24*(7), 1085-90

[37] Whitford, H. M., Alder, B. and Jones, M. (2007). A cross-sectional study of knowledge and practice of pelvic floor exercises during pregnancy and associated symptoms of stress urinary incontinence in North-East Scotland. *Midwifery, 23*(2), 204-217.

[38] Chiarelli, P. and Campbell, E. (1997). Incontinence during pregnancy. Prevalence and opportunities for continence promotion. *Aust N Z J Obstet Gynaecol, 37*(1), 66-73.

[39] Brown, S. J., Donath, S., MacArthur, C., McDonald, E. A. and Krastev, A. H. (2010). Urinary incontinence in nulliparous women before and during pregnancy: prevalence, incidence, and associated risk factors. *Int Urogynecol J, 21*(2), 193-202.

[40] Zhu, L., Li, L., Lang, J. H. and Xu, T. (2012). Prevalence and risk factors for peri- and postpartum urinary incontinence in primiparous women in China: a prospective longitudinal study. *Int Urogynecol J, 23*(5), 563-572.

[41] Liang, C. C., Chang, S. D., Lin, S. J. and Lin, Y. J. (2012). Lower urinary tract symptoms in primiparous women before and during pregnancy. *Arch Gynecol Obstet, 285*(5), 1205-1210.

[42] Sun, M. J., Chen, G. D., Chang, S. Y., Lin, K. C. and Chen, S. Y. (2005). Prevalence of lower urinary tract symptoms during pregnancy in Taiwan. *J Formos Med Assoc, 104*(3), 185-189.

[43] Sharma, J. B., Aggarwal, S., Singhal, S., Kumar, S. and Roy, K. K. (2008). Prevalence of urinary incontinence and other urological problems during pregnancy: a questionnaire based study. *Arch Gynecol Obstet, 279*(6), 845-851.

[44] Chittacharoen, A. (2005). Urinary and fecal incontinence before and during pregnancy: prevalence and associated factors. Paper presented at the 19th annual meeting of the Asian and Oceanic Congress of Obstetrics and Gynecology, Seoul, Korea, October 1-5, 2005.

[45] Abdullah, B., Ayub, S. H., Mohd Zahid, A. Z., Noorneza, A. R., Isa, M. R. and Ng, P. Y. (2008). Urinary incontinence in primigravida: the neglected pregnancy predicament. *Eur J Obstet Gynecol Reprod Biol, 198*, 110-5.

[46] Al-Mehaisen, L. M., Al-Kuran, O., Lataifeh, I. M., et al. (2009). Prevalence and frequency of severity of urinary incontinence symptoms in late pregnancy: a prospective study in the north of Jordan. Arch Gynecol Obstet, 279(4), 499-503.

[47] Erbil, N., Tas, N., Uysal, M., Kesgin, A., Kilicarslan, N. and Gokkaya, U. (2011). Urinary incontinence among pregnant Turkish women. Pak J Med Sci, 27(3), 586-590.

[48] Thomason, A. D., Miller, J. M. and Delancey, J. O. (2007). Urinary incontinence symptoms during and after pregnancy in continent and incontinent primiparas. Int Urogynecol J Pelvic Floor Dysfunct, 18(2), 147-151.

[49] Raza-Khan, F., Graziano, S., Kenton, K., Shott, S. and Brubaker, L. (2006). Peripartum urinary incontinence in a racially diverse obstetrical population. Int Urogynecol J Pelvic Floor Dysfunct, 17(5), 525-530.

[50] Oliveira, C. D, Seleme, M., Cansi, P. F., Consentino, R. F., Kumakura, F. Y., Moreira, G. A., et al. (2013). Urinary incontinence in pregnant women and its relation with socio demographic variables and quality of life. Rev Assoc Med Bras, 59(5), 460-6.

[51] Martins, G., Soler, Z. A., Cordeiro, J. A., Amaro, J. L. and Moore, K. N. (2010). Prevalence and risk factors for urinary incontinence in healthy pregnant Brazilian women. Int Urogynecol J, 21(10), 1271-1277.

[52] Adaji, S. E, Shittu, O. S., Bature, S. B., Nasir, S. and Olatunji, O. (2011). Bothersome lower urinary symptoms during pregnancy: a preliminary study using the International Consultation on Incontinence Questionnaire. Afr Health Sci, 11 Suppl 1, S46-52.

[53] Bø, K., PauckØglund, G., Sletner, L., Mørkrid, K. and Jenum, A. (2012). The prevalence of urinary incontinence in pregnancy among a multi-ethnic population resident in Norway. Br J Obstet Gynaecol, 119(11), 1354-1360.

[54] Spellacy, E. (2001). Urinary incontinence in pregnancy and the puerperium. J Obstet Gynecol Neonatal Nurs, 30(6), 634-41.

[55] Cutner, A., Cardozo, L. D. and Benness, C. J. (1991). Assessment of urinary symptoms in early pregnancy. Br J Obstet Gynaecol, 98, 1283-1286.

[56] Thorp, J. M., Norton, P. A., Wall, L. L., Kuller, J. A., Eucker, B. and Wells, E. (1999). Urinary incontinence in pregnancy and the puerperium: a prospective study. Am J Obstet Gynecol, 181, 266-273.

[57] Fritel, X., Fauconnier, A., Bader, G., et al. (2010). Diagnosis and management of adult female stress urinary incontinence: guidelines for clinical practice from the French College of Gynaecologists and Obstetricians. *Eur J Obstet Gynecol Reprod Biol*, *151*(1), 14-19.

[58] Di Stefano, M., Caserta, D., Marci, R. and Mosarini, M. (2000). Urinary incontinence in pregnancy and prevention of perineal complications of labor. *Minerva Ginecology*, *52*, 307-311.

[59] Wijma, J., Weis Potters, A. E., Tinga, D. J. and Aarnoudse, J. G. (2008). The diagnostic strength of the 24-h pad test for self-reported symptoms of urinary incontinence in pregnancy and after childbirth. *Int Urogynecol J Pelvic Floor Dysfunct*, *19*(4), 525-530.

[60] Van Kerrebroeck, P., Abrams, P., Chaikin, D., et al. (2002). The standardisation of terminology in nocturia: report from the Standardisation Sub-committee of the International Continence Society. *Neurourol Urodyn*, *21*(2), 179-183.

[61] Chaliha, C., Kalia, V., Stanton, S. L., Monga, A. and Sultan, A. H. (1999). Antenatal prediction of postpartum urinary and fecal incontinence. *Obstet Gynecol*, *94*(5 Pt 1), 689-94.

[62] Martin-Martin, S., Pascual-Fernandez, A., Alvarez-Colomo, C., Calvo-Gonzalez, R., Muñoz-Moreno, M. and Cortiñas-Gonzalez, J. R. (2014). Urinary incontinence during pregnancy and postpartum. Associated risk factors and influence of pelvic floor exercises. *Arch Esp Urol*, *67*(4), 323-30.

[63] Tanawattanacharoen, S. and Thongtawee, S. (2013). Prevalence of urinary incontinence during the late third trimester and three months postpartum period in King Chulalongkorn Memorial Hospital. *J Med Assoc Thai*, *96*(2), 144-9.

[64] Eftekhar, T., Hajibaratali, B., Ramezanzadeh, F. and Shariat, M. (2006). Postpartum evaluation of stress urinary incontinence among primiparas. *Int J Gynaecol Obstet*, *94*(2), 114-8.

[65] Lopes, D. B. M. and De Souza Praça, N. (2012). Prevalence and related factors of self-reported urinary incontinence in the postpartum period. *ACTA Paulista de Enfermagem*, *25*(4), 574-580.

[66] Hvidman, L., Foldspang, A., Mommsen, S. and Nielsen, J. B. (2003). Postpartum urinary incontinence. *Acta Obstet Gynecol Scand*, *82*(6), 556-63.

[67] Lewicky-Gaupp, C., Cao, D. C. and Culbertson, S. (2008). Urinary and anal incontinence in African American teenaged gravidas during pregnancy and the puerperium. *J Pediatr Adolesc. Gynecol*, *21*(1), 21-6.

[68] Burgio, K. L., Zyczynski, H., Locher, J. L., Richter, H. E., Redden, D. T. and Wright, K. C. (2003). Urinary incontinence in the 12-month postpartum period. *Obstet Gynecol, 102*(6), 1291-8.

[69] Pregazzi, R., Sartore, A., Troiano, L., et al. (2002). Postpartum urinary symptoms: prevalence and risk factors. *Eur J Obstet Gynecol Reprod Biol, 103*(2), 179-82.

[70] Wilson, P. D., Herbison, R. M. and Herbison, G. P. (1996). Obstetric practice and the prevalence of urinary incontinence three months after delivery. *Br J Obstet Gynaecol, 103*(2), 154-61.

[71] Boyles, S. H., Li, H., Mori, T., Osterweil, P. and Guise, J. M. (2009). Effect of mode of delivery on the incidence of urinary incontinence in primiparous women. *Obstet Gynecol, 113*(1), 134-41.

[72] Baydock, S. A., Flood, C., Schulz, J. A., et al. (2009). Prevalence and risk factors for urinary and fecal incontinence four months after vaginal delivery. *J Obstet Gynaecol Can, 31*(1), 36-41.

[73] Gartland, D., Donath, S., MacArthur, C. and Brown, S. J. (2012). The onset, recurrence and associated obstetric risk factors for urinary incontinence in the first 18 months after a first birth: an Australian nulliparous cohort study. *Br J Obstet Gynaecol, 119*(11), 1361-9.

[74] Quiboeuf, E., Saurel-Cubizolles, M. J., Fritel, X. and EDEN Mother-Child Cohort Study Group. (2016). Trends in urinary incontinence in women between 4 and 24 months postpartum in the EDEN cohort. *Br J Obstet Gynaecol, 123*(7), 1222-8.

[75] Wesnes, S. L., Hunskaar, S., Bo, K. and Rortveit G. (2009). The effect of urinary incontinence status during pregnancy and delivery mode on incontinence postpartum. A cohort study. *Br J Obstet Gynaecol, 116*(5), 700-7.

[76] Hatem, M., Pasquier, J. C., Fraser, W. and Lepire E. (2007). Factors associated with postpartum urinary/anal incontinence in primiparous women in Quebec. *J Obstet Gynaecol Can, 29*(3), 232-9.

[77] Hansen, B. B, Svare, J., Viktrup, L., Jørgensen, T. and Lose, G. (2012). Urinary incontinence during pregnancy and 1 year after delivery in primiparous women compared with a control group of nulliparous women. *Neurourol Urodyn, 31*(4), 475-80.

[78] Chang, S. R., Chen, K. H., Lin, H. H., Lin, M. I., Chang, T. C. and Lin, W. A. (2014). Association of mode of delivery with urinary incontinence and changes in urinary incontinence over the first year postpartum. *Obstet Gynecol, 123*(3), 568-77.

[79] Diez-Itza, I., Arrue, M., Ibañez, L., Murgiondo, A., Paredes, J. and Sarasqueta, C. (2010). Factors involved in stress urinary incontinence 1 year after first delivery. *Int Urogynecol J*, *21*(4), 439-45.

[80] Brown, S., Gartland, D., Perlen, S., McDonald, E. and MacArthur, C. (2015). Consultation about urinary and faecal incontinence in the year after childbirth: a cohort study. *Br J Obstet Gynaecol*, *122*(7), 954-62.

[81] Chan, S. S., Cheung, R. Y., Yiu, K. W., Lee, L. L. and Chung, T. K. (2013). Prevalence of urinary and fecal incontinence in Chinese women during and after their first pregnancy. *Int Urogynecol J*, *24*(9), 1473-9.

[82] Barbosa, A. M., Marini, G., Piculo, F., Rudge, C. V., Calderon, I. M. and Rudge, M. V. (2013). Prevalence of urinary incontinence and pelvic floor muscle dysfunction in primiparae two years after cesarean section: cross-sectional study. *Sao Paulo Med J*, *131*(2), 95-9.

[83] Herrmann, V., Scarpa, K., Palma, P. C. and Riccetto, C. Z. (2009). Stress urinary incontinence 3 years after pregnancy: correlation to mode of delivery and parity. *Int Urogynecol J Pelvic Floor Dysfunct*, *20*(3), 281-8.

[84] Gartland, D., MacArthur, C., Woolhouse, H., McDonald, E. and Brown, S. (2016). Frequency, severity and risk factors for urinary and faecal incontinence at 4 years postpartum: a prospective cohort. *Br J Obstet Gynaecol*, *123*(7), 1203-11.

[85] Fritel, X., Khoshnood, B. and Fauconnier, A. (2013). Specific obstetrical risk factors for urinary versus anal incontinence 4 years after first delivery. *Prog Urol*, *23*(11), 911-6.

[86] Liang, C. C., Wu, M. P., Lin, S. J., Lin, Y. J., Chang, S. D. and Wang, H. H. (2013). Clinical impact of and contributing factors to urinary incontinence in women 5 years after first delivery. *Int Urogynecol J*, *24*(1), 99-104.

[87] MacArthur, C., Glazener, C. M., Wilson, P. D., Lancashire, R. J, Herbison, G. P. and Grant, A. M. (2006). Persistent urinary incontinence and delivery mode history: a six-year longitudinal study. *Br J Obstet Gynaecol*, *113*(2), 218-24.

[88] Viktrup, L., Rortveit, G. and Lose, G. (2006). Risk of stress urinary incontinence twelve years after the first pregnancy and delivery. *Obstet Gynecol*, *108*(2), 248-54.

[89] MacArthur, C., Wilson, D., Herbison, P., Lancashire, R. J, Hagen, S., Toozs-Hobson, P., et al. (2016). Urinary incontinence persisting after childbirth: extent, delivery history, and effects in a 12-year longitudinal cohort study. *Br J Obstet Gynaecol, 123*(6), 1022-9.

[90] Gyhagen, M., Bullarbo, M., Nielsen, T. F. and Milsom, I. (2013). Prevalence and risk factors for pelvic organ prolapse 20 years after childbirth: a national cohort study in singleton primiparae after vaginal or caesarean delivery. *Br J Obstet Gynaecol, 120*(2), 152-60.

In: Urinary Incontinence
Editor: Debra Newton

ISBN: 978-1-53610-099-0
© 2016 Nova Science Publishers, Inc.

Chapter 2

RISK FACTORS FOR THE DEVELOPMENT OF POSTPARTUM URINARY INCONTINENCE IN PRIMIPAROUS WOMEN

Bussara Sangsawang[1,], Nucharee Sangsawang[1] and Denchai Laiwattana[2]*
[1]Department of Maternal–Child Nursing and Midwifery Nursing, Faculty of Nursing, Srinakharinwirot University, Thailand
[2]Department of Neurosurgery, Bangkok Hospital Trat, Trat, Thailand

ABSTRACT

Urinary incontinence (UI), the complaint of involuntary loss of urine, is a common condition during the immediate postpartum period after a woman's first pregnancy. The prevalence of UI is high and approximately 18.96% to 55.9% of all pregnant women develop UI during pregnancy. During the postpartum period, the prevalence of UI ranges from 6.9% to 47.0%, which is lower when compared with the prevalence during the third trimester of pregnancy. However the remission rate of UI at three months after childbirth as high as 86.4%.

UI is a serious health problem during the postpartum period that affects the quality of life (QoL) of postpartum women by disrupting the women's daily activities. Postpartum women who have UI feel frustrated and embarrassed.

* Corresponding author: twinnui@hotmail.com.

It is well known that UI is related to the weakening of the pelvic floor muscle (PFM), connective tissue and fascia as well as their supportive and sphincteric function. The pathophysiology of UI is multifactorial but there is a lot of evidence to support the critical role of pregnancy and vaginal delivery in the development of UI. Pregnancy may be associated with a reduction in PFM strength that can develop into UI. In addition to pregnancy itself, the physiological changes associated with the second stage of labor can cause significant stress on the PFM appear to play a role in postpartum UI. However, the exact causes of postpartum UI remain unclear.

Several risk factors have been proven to be associated with UI, some of which are potentially modifiable to facilitate early intervention for target at risk women. Aging is an important role in UI development in the form of genetic risk factors. The other significant modifiable risk factors for postpartum UI include high body mass index, obesity, smoking, constipation, multiparity, UI before pregnancy, UI during pregnancy, prolonged second stage of labor, mode of delivery and neonatal birth weight. Antenatal UI increases the risk for postpartum incontinence, which in turn increases the risk for long–term persistent UI. The second stage of labor has modest effects on postpartum PFM function. After their first delivery, women who deliver vaginally have a higher incidence of postpartum SUI than those who deliver by cesarean section (C/S). Postpartum women who have higher BMI and weight retention at six months postpartum are at increased risk for postpartum UI.

In decreasing the risk for postpartum UI, pregnant women who perform pelvic floor muscle exercises (PFME) may be able to prevent postpartum UI. Postpartum weight loss by advice about eating and exercise habits to avoid weight retention after delivery can also decrease the risk for UI and restore the continence mechanism at six months postpartum. Moreover, elective cesarean sections in these women also have a preventive effect and lower the risk for developing postpartum UI.

The purpose of this review chapter is to identify the risk factors for the development of UI in postpartum women. This understanding can be useful for health professionals in educating and counseling pregnant and postpartum women about preventing and reducing the risk factors contributing to the development of UI during postpartum period.

INTRODUCTION

Urinary incontinence (UI), a common condition during the immediate postpartum period after a woman's first pregnancy is defined by the

International Continence Society (ICS) as the complaint of involuntary loss of urine [1].

Urinary incontinence is a serious health problem during the postpartum period that affects the quality of life (QoL) of postpartum women by disrupting the women's daily activities [2]. Postpartum women who have UI are associated with feelings of frustration and embarrassment, in addition, the postpartum women report that diminished their ability to have sexual relations and reduced involvement in physical and recreational activities [3]. Women with UI during pregnancy and childbirth have a worse QoL than continent women [4]. Furthermore, the prevalence of depressive symptoms is also higher in women with UI that those without UI. Women who have UI after delivery are more likely to develop postpartum depression than those without UI [5]. Interestingly, postpartum UI not only develops postpartum depression, but also develops anxiety after delivery [6]. In prospective cohort study, Goyeneche et al. [6] also found that UI was associated with anxiety in the postpartum period. Moreover, women who have UI during pregnancy or postpartum period have significant risk factors for increasing UI later in life [7].

The prevalence of UI is high at approximately 18.96% [8] to 55.9% [9] of all pregnant women. During the postpartum period, the prevalence of UI ranges from 6.9% [10] to 47.0% [11], which is lower when compared with the prevalence during the third trimester of pregnancy. However, the remission rate of UI at three months after childbirth is high at up to 86.4% [12].

Many aspects of UI pathophysiology remain uncertain. The mechanism of UI is due to the fact that bladder pressure remains lower than urethral closure pressure, and UI may result from bladder or urethral impairment. When urethral closure pressure is lower than bladder pressure, leakage occurs [13].

Urethral mobility increases during pregnancy [14]. It would be interesting to learn whether or not greater mobility is associated with a higher risk for SUI during pregnancy [13]. There exists a link between heightened prenatal urethral mobility and postnatal SUI [15]. Urethral closure pressure and sphincter volume diminish after childbirth [16, 17]. Urethral closure pressure is lower in primiparous stress incontinent women than in primiparous continent women [18].

Pregnancy and delivery are significant risk factors for the development of UI in young women [19, 20]. Pregnancy may be associated with the reduction of pelvic floor muscle strength which can develop SUI [21]. However, the exact mechanism of pregnancy–related SUI is not well understood [22]. Commonly encountered prenatal physiological changes such as increasing pressure of the growing uterus and fetal weight on pelvic floor muscle throughout pregnancy, together with pregnancy–related hormonal changes in progesterone, estrogen and relaxin, may lead to reduced strength and supportive and sphincteric function of pelvic floor muscle [23]. Pelvic floor muscle weakness causes bladder–neck and urethral mobility leading to urethral sphincter incompetence. Hence, when intra–abdominal pressure is increased, the pressure inside the bladder becomes greater than the urethral closure pressure and the urethral sphincter is not strong enough to maintain urethral closure. Urinary leakage is the result [23].

Similar to UI during pregnancy, postpartum UI may be explained by a deficiency in urethral closure resistance and pelvic floor muscle trauma associated with vaginal delivery [13, 24]. Urinary incontinence during the postpartum period is essentially associated with pregnancy and delivery [25]. Regardless, many aspects of the pathophysiology of postpartum incontinence remain poorly understood [13].

During labor and delivery, the descent of the fetus through the pelvic cavity causes great trauma to pelvic organs, notably in the lower urinary tract and its supporting structures, which could cause lower urinary symptoms during the postnatal period [26]. It is common knowledge that vaginal delivery or childbirth–related pelvic floor trauma causes a significant stretching of muscular, fascial and ligamentous supports of the pelvic floor structures with consequent loss of support of the bladder neck and urethra, which plays a significant role in the pathogenesis of UI [24, 27, 28]. Moreover, induced labor may create greater mechanical forces on the pelvic floor muscles and nerves resulting in greater stretching of these structures [24]. Therefore, it is likely that the pathogenesis of postpartum UI includes not only the effects of pelvic floor trauma on urethrovesical hypermobility under stress, but also a deficiency in urethral resistance [24].

In particular, UI is common during pregnancy and the puerperium period. Urinary incontinence prevalence peaks at the end of pregnancy. After delivery, the prevalence of UI diminishes during the postpartum period [13] and resolves itself in the vast majority of cases [29]. Quiboeut et al. found UI remission to occur in half all cases between 4 and 24 months postpartum [25]. The remission rate observed during the postpartum period is higher among women with caesarean deliveries [25]. The healing process may take some time after delivery [30]. In primiparous women, UI symptoms tend to resolve within 3 months after delivery [31]. However, this remission is not complete at 3–4 months and can continue for a long time in the absence of an intercurrent obstetric event for up to at least 24 months postpartum [25]. Viktrup et al. found the highest prevalence to occur just before delivery with a sudden drop and progressive remission at twelve months after first delivery [29]. Therefore, UI is a dynamic process that may sometimes begin before first delivery and disappear during the year following delivery [32].

Despite this clear association, the mechanism involved with UI during pregnancy and the postpartum period remains unclear. Similarly, the pathophysiology of the development of UI is not clearly understood. However, it has been suggested that UI could be caused by both hormonal and mechanical changes occurring during this period [33, 34]. This effect of pregnancy on UI may persist after delivery, but is likely to be spontaneously reversible more often or more rapidly after a caesarean than a vaginal delivery [25]. After pregnancy, most women recover their prepregnancy hormonal levels, and the pressure of the enlarged uterus on the bladder and pelvic floor muscle resolves. Postnatal remission of UI may be explained by the resolution of hormonal and metabolic changes associated with pregnancy and spontaneous healing of traumatic lesions due to vaginal childbirth [13].

In general, UI can affect 27.4% of parous women for 6 months postpartum with only a small portion of women experiencing spontaneous resolution [35]. Thomason et al. [36] found that only 8% of pregnant women who developed UI during pregnancy had resolution, but in 47% of those who had UI, incontinence had not resolved at 6 months postpartum. Continence appears to be restored more frequently in women with caesarean deliveries whereas vaginal delivery appears to expose women to a relapse or longer recovery [25].

The purpose of this review chapter is to identify the risk factors for the development of UI in postpartum women. The understanding gained can be useful for health professions to educate and counsel pregnant and postpartum women in preventing and reducing the risk factors contributing to the development of UI during the postpartum period.

FACTORS INCREASING THE RISK FOR POSTPARTUM URINARY INCONTINENCE IN PRIMIPAROUS WOMEN

The following section discusses the risk factors for the development of postpartum UI in primiparous women. Understanding of this topic can be useful for health professionals in informing and counseling both pregnant and postpartum women to prevent and reduce the risk factors contributing to the development of UI during pregnancy and the postpartum period.

Multiple factors have been found to be associated with the development of postpartum UI, including the following:

1. Maternal Age

Maternal age is one of the most important and well–known risk factors for pelvic floor dysfunction. Maternal age is also considered the only non-modifiable risk factor that is inherently and directly related to the incidence of stress urinary incontinence (SUI) and pelvic organ prolapsed (POP) [37–42].

Stress urinary incontinence during pregnancy and the postpartum period is associated with advanced maternal age [43, 44]. In fact, the main risk factor for postpartum UI is maternal age [12]. Zhu et al. [45] reported the risk for SUI incidence to increase with maternal age (OR 1.041, 95% CI 1.027–1.055). MacArthur et al. [46] found older maternal age to be significantly associated with increased risk for persistent or long-term UI. Cerruto et al. [12] found the prevalence of UI to increase with increasing age and a significant risk factor for UI in pregnancy to be maternal age >35 years.

These findings are supported by Glazener et al. [47] who found maternal age to be an independent risk factor for new onset of UI with increased risk for older women at 35 years and over. This finding is significant evidence emphasizing the role of maternal age at the time of first pregnancy as an independent risk factor for the occurrence of UI [48]. Hvidman et al. [34] found pregnant women aged 30 years and older to be at significantly greater risk for SUI than younger women (OR = 1.4). This finding was also supported by Groutz et al. [49] who reported that older maternal aged over 30 years at first birth also constituted a significant risk factor for persistent and long–term UI.

Older age at first delivery may be a risk factor for pelvic floor trauma [50] in older pregnant women because advanced maternal age leads to loss of nerve function and urethral closure pressure [51] in addition to decreases in the total number of striated muscle fibers of the urethral sphincter at a rate of 2% a year [52, 53]. The effects of age may be attributed to the weakening of supporting pelvic structures and nerves associated with the aging process [54, 55]. Furthermore, older maternal age before first pregnancy is a contributing factor affecting the degree of injury to the pelvic floor muscles [56]. Trowbridge et al. [57] conducted a cohort study to evaluate the effects of aging on urethral support, urethral function and levator function in 82 nulliparous women. According to the findings, increasing age was associated with decreasing maximal urethral closure pressure (r = –0.758, P < .001); however, pelvic organ support, urethral support and levator function were not found to change with increasing age.

In contrast, few studies show the association between women with younger age and UI. In this follow–up study of a large Norwegian EI survey, Ebbesen et al. found increases in age to be associated with reduced incidence and remission of UI. Both incidence and remission of UI were found to be highest in women at 20 – 39 years of age [58]. Hojberg et al. [59] reported that younger pregnant women aged between 15 to 24 years had a significantly higher risk for UI than those aged between 25 to 29 years (OR = 1.5; 95% CI 1.0–2.4). Furthermore, Lewicky–Gaupp et al. [60] determined the prevalence of UI during pregnancy in adolescent African–American women, finding a high prevalence of UI in adolescent pregnant women during the third trimester at 43%.

2. Parity

Parity is one of the most reliable predictors for developing UI and POP [61] and an established risk factor for SUI among young and middle–aged women [62]. Regardless, the underlying etiology is not completely understood. MacArthur et al. [46] found an association between persistent incontinence and increasing number of child births. The aforementioned findings are similar other studies that also found higher prevalence of UI to be associated with greater parity [63–65]. It is common knowledge that childbirth–related pelvic floor trauma with consequent reductions in pelvic floor muscle strength and loss of support of the bladder neck and urethra play a significant role in the pathogenesis of UI. Özdemır et al. [66] compared pelvic floor muscle strength in women who had had 1–3, 4–6, and more than 6 deliveries, reporting the highest pelvic floor muscle strength to be found in women who had 1–3 deliveries.

Furthermore, pelvic floor muscle strength decreased as the number of deliveries increased. It is evident, therefore, that the pelvic floor damage taking place during pregnancy, labor and delivery may be involved. Pregnant women suffer from a variety of mechanical and hormonal changes that have been linked to UI. In addition, the passage of the newborn through the birth canal causes injuries to the structures of the pelvic floor that can also modify the continence mechanism. Some data also suggests that constitutional variables may predispose women to UI after childbirth [67].

Pregazzia et al. [24] reported that UI appears to be associated with general maternal factors such as parity (P < .001) and induced labor with prostaglandins (P < .018). Interestingly, the pathogenesis of postpartum UI can be concluded to include not only the effects of pelvic floor trauma on urethrovesical mobility under stress, but also a deficiency in urethral resistance caused by drugs such as prostaglandins. Arrue et al. [33] suggested that the mechanism causing the association between parity and UI might be related to the hormonal changes occurring during gestation.

The number of previous pregnancies and deliveries is significantly higher in incontinent pregnant women than continent pregnant women [68]. Primiparae who deliver vaginally are also at a significantly higher risk for UI than nulliparae. Furthermore, multiparous women are associated with greater risk for UI than primiparae [59, 69]. A study by Pregazzia et al. [24] reported 20% of multiparae to present with UI with a rate of 8.2% in primiparae (P < .0001). Urge urinary incontinence (UUI) has been found to be present in 13% of multiparae and in 5.5% of primiparae (P < .004). Marshall et al. [70] reported a high reverse association in percentage of UI and parity at 68% in multiparous women who had given birth five times or more as compared to 66% in multiparous women who had given birth 2–4 times and 55.0% for primigravidae.

This finding was supported by Wesnes et al. [43] who investigated the associated risk factors for UI during pregnancy among 43,279 pregnant women, finding parity to be a strong and significant risk factor for incontinence in adjusted analyses both before pregnancy (odds ratio [OR] 2.5, 95% confidence interval [CI] 2.4–2.7 for primiparous women and OR 3.3, 95% CI 3.1–3.5 for multiparous women) and during pregnancy (ORs 2.0, 95% CI 1.9–2.1 and 2.1, 95% CI 2.0–2.2, respectively).

3. Mode of Delivery

Pregnancy and vaginal delivery are major risk factors for weakened pelvic floor muscle, which can cause SUI and POP in younger women. The aforementioned conditions can have negative consequences on sexual, physical and professional activities [71]. In the processes of pregnancy and childbirth, chronic fetal oppression of the pelvic floor musculature and innervation of the supporting tissues of the pelvic cavity can injure the pelvic floor muscles and cause urethral sphincter denervation damage; the fetus passing through the soft birth canal can also directly damage the pelvic floor, anal sphincter and perineum [72–74]. Thus, vaginal delivery is associated with damage to the pelvic floor muscles and nerves, and this damage is thought to be increased with the number of vaginal deliveries and duration of the second stage of labor [54]. In addition to pregnancy itself, the physiological changes associated with the second stage of labor appear to play a role in postpartum UI. In women who deliver by vaginal birth, a prolonged second stage of labor has been found to be associated with significantly higher odds for postpartum incontinence [75].

Vaginal delivery is associated with pelvic floor dysfunction and reduced urethral closure pressure. Furthermore, bladder neck mobility is increased significantly after all vaginal births [76]. These changes are caused by traction or stretching of the pudendal nerve fibers that supply the pelvic floor muscles [48, 77–79]. A normal vaginal delivery causes significant strain on the pelvic floor and can result in some women of fertile age developing UI [80]. Tunn et al. [81] suggested that vaginal childbirth results in neuromuscular and ischemic damage to the bladder outlet and urethra, thereby increasing the risk for postpartum UI. The second stage of labor has a modest effect on postpartum pelvic floor function [82].

The damage to pelvic floor musculature, fascial support and nerve supply usually occurs during the second stage of labor when the mother pushes and the fetal head distends and stretches the pelvic floor [48]. Peschers et al. [83] used palpation, perineometry, and perineal ultrasound 3–8 days after delivery to evaluate the pelvic floor muscle strength values of primiparous and multiparous women who had vaginal deliveries. Their study showed that the pelvic floor muscle strength decreased significantly after vaginal delivery. Therefore, vaginal delivery increases the short–term risk for UI in young and middle–aged women more than cesarean delivery [84].

Numerous studies have reported the impact of the mode of delivery on the development of UI in women, comparing the effects of caesarean section and vaginal delivery. The largest study carried out in an Italian population by Torrisi et al. [85] confirmed that vaginal delivery is a strong important risk factor for the development of UI (OR 3.3, CI 2.0–5.3, $p < .001$). In a population–based cohort study by Leijonhufvud et al. [86], the researchers estimated the risk for UI related to vaginal birth or cesarean delivery in 60,122 women with vaginal delivery and 30,880 women with cesarean delivery. According to the findings, there was a significantly increased risk for UI later in life among the women who had delivered only by vaginal childbirth compared to those having only cesarean deliveries.

In Canada, Farrell et al. [87] found the incidence of UI at 6 months postpartum in women who had undergone vaginal delivery to be 26%, including obvious clinical symptoms in 4% of patients. Meanwhile, the UI rate in women who had undergone cesarean section was 10%. Nygaard [84] found women who had delivered vaginally have two–fold more incontinence the first delivery than those delivered by cesarean section. In addition, vaginal delivery is an even greater risk factor for long–term UI after delivery than caesarean section.

Gyhagen et al. [88] conducted a study in women 20 years after delivery to examine the effects of one vaginal delivery (VD) compared with one caesarean section (CS) on the prevalence, severity and discomfort of UI subtypes—SUI, UUI and mixed urinary incontinence (MUI) at 20 years after delivery. According to the findings, the prevalence rates of SUI, UUI and MUI were found to be 15.3, 6.1, 14.4%, respectively, and were higher for all subtypes after VD versus CS. Furthermore, the severity of UI differs with mode of delivery whereby moderate to severe incontinence symptoms have been found to more prevalent after VD (21.3%) compared with CS (13.5%; adj OR 1.68, 95% confidence interval [95% CI] 1.40–2.03). The aforementioned study concluded that the prevalence rates of SUI, UUI and MUI were higher for moderate to severe UI and UI discomfort was reported more frequently after VD than CS at 20 years after one delivery.

Vaginal delivery presents an even greater risk factor for POP [80]. Rogers et al. [82] found greater decent of the anterior vaginal wall in women delivering by vaginal birth. Primiparae who deliver vaginally are also at significantly higher risk for SUI than nulliparae (OR 5.9; 95% CI 4.1–8.3). Furthermore, multiparous women are associated with greater risk for SUI than primiparae [59, 69]. A study by Marshall et al. [70] reported a high percentage of UI at approximately 68% in multiparous women who had given birth five times or more as compared to 66% in multiparous women who had given birth 2–4 times and 55.0% for primigravidae.

Urinary incontinence is commonly found in women with instrumental delivery compared to spontaneous vaginal delivery (36% and 34%, respectively), and lowest in women with elective cesarean section (13%) [89]. These results are consistent with the study of Arya et al. [90] who found forceps delivery to be associated with higher risk for UI compared with spontaneous vaginal delivery. Forceps delivery causes more stretching which damages the nerves and connective tissues of the pelvic floor. The increased incidence of UI associated with forceps delivery may be related to the accelerated descent of the fetal head by forceps extraction as compared to normal labor [91].

In addition, Yang et al. [92] found an increase in the prevalence of UI after forceps delivery compared to vaginal delivery, assessing 1,889 primiparous postpartum women and finding UI prevalence to be related to vaginal delivery (OR 5.42, 95% CI 2.60–11.32, p = 0.000) and forceps delivery (OR 7.0, 95% CI 2.40–20.41, p = 0.000). Based on the findings, vaginal delivery has a risk for impact on UI in postpartum women, especially in cases involving forceps delivery. For vacuum extraction, the effects of assisted vaginal delivery may be also explained by the fact that vacuum delivery requires extra mechanical forces acting on the baby along the genital tract, which may cause damage to the pelvic floor support and anal sphincter [54]. In contrast, MacArthur et al. [46] found no statistically significant associations between persistent or long-term UI and forceps or vacuum extraction delivery. They found no evidence of any association between persistent or long–term UI and forceps or vacuum extraction delivery. According to the findings, Arrue et al. [33] found no statistically significant association between the mode of vaginal delivery and UI at 6 months after delivery. Li et al. [93] found the delivery modes to not differ significantly with respect to the incidence of postpartum UI or pelvic muscle floor muscle strength.

Although childbirth is well–documented as a major risk factor for UI, delivery by caesarean section provides protection [46]. Caesarean delivery (CD) reduces the risk for pelvic floor dysfunction following delivery, including UI, anal incontinence (AI), POP and pelvic pain in addition to preserving sexual function [86, 94, 95]. Moreover, cesarean section and pelvic floor rehabilitation have a protective effect on preventing the development of POP [61]. In addition, women who have undergone CD are more likely to report lower sexual function scores than women who delivered vaginally [82].

In the western world and most high–income countries, the incidence of caesarean section on maternal requests for non–medical reasons is steadily rising [96]. Women and healthcare providers frequently report prevention of pelvic floor dysfunction as one of the main reasons for elective caesarean section [97] because prolapse seems to be a risk factor for UI and UI > 10 years. Therefore, women with sPOP after vaginal delivery fare significantly worse than women with sPOP after caesarean section [41].

Cesarean section could have a protective role in postpartum UI in comparison with vaginal delivery [98, 99]. Women with cesarean sections are at lower risk for postpartum UI than those with vaginal deliveries [100]. This finding is supported by Boyles et al. [101] who reported that cesarean section reduced the risk for postpartum UI and found pregnant women who had had vaginal deliveries to be more likely to have UI than women who had cesarean deliveries (odds ratio of 4.96 [95% confidence interval 3.82–6.44], P<.001). At 6 weeks postpartum, Farrel et al. [87] reported UI in 35% of 115 women who delivered by forceps, 23% of 333 women after vaginal delivery, 9% of 98 women after cesarean during labor and 4% of women after cesarean before labor. Mason et al. [102] found no differences in UI prevalence in women at 8 weeks postpartum categorized by type of cesarean (16% after "planned cesarean" versus 17% after "emergency cesarean"), even though the women who delivered by cesarean section had fewer UI than those who delivered vaginally without instrumentation (35%).

Goldberg et al. [103] reported that women delivering vaginally demonstrated a significantly higher rate of SUI than women delivering by cesarean section (OR 2.28, CI 1.14–4.55, $p < 0.019$). Fritel et al. [13] reported cesarean delivery to be associated with lower rates of SUI than vaginal delivery. Rørtveit et al. [80] found the prevalence of UI and POP to be lower in women delivering solely by caesarean section than in those who have delivered vaginally. Of the women's pre–pregnancy continence, Brown et al. [75] found 26% of women to report new incontinence at 3 months postpartum. Compared with women who had had a spontaneous vaginal birth, women who had had a caesarean section before labor (adjusted odds ratio [OR] 0.2, 95% CI 0.1–0.5) or in the first stage of labor (adjusted OR 0.2, 95% CI 0.1–0.4) were less likely to be incontinent at 3 months postpartum. In 3,405 primiparous women at 3 months postpartum, Glazener et al. [47], found the women who delivered by cesarean section to have decreased prevalence and incidence of UI (16% and 7%, respectively) compared with those who delivered vaginally without instrumentation (30% and 18%, respectively). Chaliha et al. [104] conducted a cohort study finding SUI to have increased in 130 women at 3 months after vaginal delivery compared with 31 women who had delivered by cesarean section (21% versus 13%, respectively). However, there were no differences in UUI (5% versus 3%) or urgency (15% versus 10%). In another cohort study, Eason et al. [105] conducted a cohort study in 949 women. They found 12% of primiparae who delivered by cesarean section to have UI at 3 months compared with 31% who had delivered vaginally.

MacArthur et al. [46] found the risk for persistent and long–term UI to be significantly lower following caesarean section deliveries but not following a subsequent vaginal birth. At 1 year postpartum, Schytt et al. [7] found the prevalence of SUI to be greater in women who underwent vaginal delivery (23.4%) than cesarean delivery (10.6%). Groutz et al. [106] found the prevalence of UI at 1 year after delivery to be similar between vaginal delivery and cesarean delivery for obstructed labor (10.3% and 12.0%, respectively), but lower after cesarean delivery before labor (3.4%).

Women who have had a caesarean section before the onset of labor or in the first stage of labor are significantly less likely to report UI after the birth compared with women who have had a spontaneous vaginal birth. Brown et al. [75] found prolonged second stage labor to be associated with increased likelihood for postpartum incontinence in women with spontaneous vaginal births (adjusted OR 1.9, 95% CI 1.1–3.4) or operative vaginal births (adjusted OR 1.7, 95% CI 1.0–2.8).

Overall, the research indicates that caesarean section may protect against UI in women of fertile age, but the effect does not persist when the women become older when the prevalence of incontinence is highest [80].

In contrast, cesarean section is not associated with a major reduction in UI [107], which concurs with the findings of Chou et al. [108] who reported cesarean section to not prevent SUI in primiparous mothers at 1 year postpartum. Cesarean section is reported to reduce the incidence of postpartum UI by 5–10% and has a protective effect on early postpartum POP. Li et al. [93] found the incidence of UI in the cesarean section group to be 9.09%, which was lower than that of 16.87% for the normal delivery group. However, the difference was not statistically significant (P > 0.05). At the same time, incidence of POP in the cesarean section group was 53.03%, which is significantly lower than 86.75% in the vaginal delivery group (P < 0.05). At 1 year after delivery, Groutz et al. [106] found the incidence of UI in women who had undergone cesarean section and vaginal delivery to be 10.3–12% at 1 year postpartum. In addition, the incidence of UI in the cesarean section group was lower than that in the vaginal delivery group, but the difference was not statistically significant. The insignificance of the aforementioned finding indicates that cesarean section does not reduce the incidence of postpartum UI.

As previously mentioned, the results of some studies [93, 106] showed the incidence of postpartum UI and pelvic floor muscle strength to not differ significantly between different delivery modes. Therefore, the idea of pregnant women undergoing cesarean section requires additional consideration. Similarly, Wesnes and Lose [109] suggested that cesarean section cannot be recommended (evidence grade D) to prevent UI during pregnancy and postpartum. In other words, if lifestyle recommendations are addressed in association with pregnancy, the incidence of UI during pregnancy and the postpartum period is likely to decrease.

4. Obesity, High Body Mass Index (BMI) and High Weight Gain During Pregnancy

Obesity is another established causal factor of UI and POP [61]. Increased body mass index (BMI) before pregnancy has been found to be associated with an increased risk for developing UI and appears to be linear in that the higher the BMI, the greater the risk for developing incontinence [110]. Therefore, excessive weight gain during pregnancy also increases the risk for UI during pregnancy and the postpartum period, but this relationship is inconclusive [111, 112]. It can be concluded, therefore, that women who are overweight or obese (BMI > 25) at the start of pregnancy tend to retain more postpartum weight [113–115].

Although the effects of obesity on postpartum SUI are remain unclear, it seems that a high BMI during pregnancy may worsen pelvic floor weakness beginning during pregnancy and after vaginal delivery [116]. In addition, high weight gain during pregnancy also increases the risk for subsequent pelvic floor muscle dysfunction. Barbosa et al. [117] found higher weight gain during pregnancy to be associated with an increased risk for postpartum pelvic floor muscle dysfunction (OR = 1.3 and 95% CI = 1.1–1.4 for digital palpation; OR = 1.2 and 95% CI = 1.0–1.3 for perineometry). This finding might be explained in that the physiological weight gain during pregnancy may lead to increased pressure on the PFM and bladder possibly leading to greater urethral mobility [24,118]. Moreover, obesity may impair blood flow and nerve innervation to the bladder and urethra [119] whereby increased BMI is correlated with increased intra–abdominal pressure during urodynamic assessments and increased the risk for SUI later in life [118, 120].

Similarly, the effects of neonatal birth weight may also be linked to the association between fetal macrosomia and prolonged second stage of labor [55] with consequent increased risk for injury to the pelvic floor musculature and nerves. The effects of high birth weight are seen in the extra weight borne by the lower abdominal organs during pregnancy in addition to the size of the infant passing through the delivery canal [117]. Therefore, the first child's weight is already known to be a risk factor for UI after the first delivery [121, 122]. Pizzoferrato et al. [32] found an increase of 100 g in the first child's weight to increase the risk for long-term incontinence. The association between the first child's weight and risk for UI can also be explained by metabolic causes, e.g., gestational diabetes mellitus (GDM). Similarly, Eftekhar et al. study [100] found the prevalence of UI to be associated with high birth weight (P = 0.00, $\chi2$ = 25.5).

Obesity and overweight during pregnancy are risk factors for an increased risk for UI during pregnancy and the postpartum period found in numerous studies. In the study of Hojberg et al. [59] it was reported that pregnant women with pre–pregnancy BMI of more than 30 kg/m^2 and 35 kg/m^2 were at significantly higher risk for SUI than those with a normal pre-pregnancy BMI (OR = 1.7; 95% CI 0.9–3.2 and OR = 2.5; 95% CI 1.0–6.0, respectively). Similarly, Liang et al. [123] reported women with a pre–pregnancy BMI of more than 30 kg/m^2 to be at increased risk for developing SUI during pregnancy. Brown et al. [9] reported that pregnant women with a BMI 30 kg/m^2 or more were at increased risk for developing de novo UI during pregnancy (AdjOR = 1.5, 95% CI 1.0–2.3).

Hvidman et al. [34] found pregnant women with a pre-pregnancy BMI of more than 30 kg/m^2 to be associated with a high rate of SUI (OR = 2.2). Diez–Itza et al. [111] found the women at term pregnancy with at term body weight of 75 kg or more to have more than doubled the risk for SUI. These findings are similar to the study of Arrue et al. [33] who reported continent primigravida women who had higher weight gains in pregnancy to have increased the risk for SUI after delivery.

Several studies have shown the association between obesity and postpartum SUI. High BMI and weight retention following childbirth increase the risk for postpartum UI. Ruiz de Viñaspre Hernández et al. [113] found that high BMI and weight retention at six months postpartum increase the risk for postpartum UI. Glazener et al. [47] indicated the persistence of pregnancy–related UI during the postpartum period to be associated with higher maternal BMI > 25 before pregnancy (OR 1.68, 95%; CI 1.12-2.43).

Higher maternal BMI during pregnancy may play a role in the link between pregnancy and long–term postpartum SUI. Yang et al. [92], found an association between SUI at 6 months after delivery and higher maternal weight at term. Svare et al. [116] reported a BMI ≥ 30 kg/m^2 to be marginally associated with UI at 1 year after delivery. This is a similar to Arrue et al. [124] who found a higher BMI in pregnant women at term to be the only independent risk factor for the persistence of SUI at 2 years postpartum (OR 1.19; 95%; confidence interval 1.08–1.32). However, the mechanism increasing BMI that favors the presence of SUI during pregnancy and its persistence at 2 years postpartum remains unknown.

Pizzoferrato et al. [32] found the factors associated with UI at 12 years after first pregnancy to be high BMI (OR = 1.17; 95%; CI: 1.04–1.32, by 1 kg/m2), thereby increasing BMI (OR = 1.43; 95%; CI: 1.19–1.73) with higher fetal or newborn weight (OR = 1.08 95%; CI: 1.001–1.16, by 100 g). Subak et al. [125] concluded that the risk for UI in childbearing women increases between 7% and 12% per unit increase in BMI. This is a similar to Ruiz de Viñaspre Hernández's study [113], which found the risk for UI to increase by 9% per unit increase in BMI, or 8% when the effects of other variables are taken into account. Similar findings were also reported by Rodríguez–Mias et al. [61], who found the average BMIs in the SUI and POP groups to be 28 and 26.6, respectively. Moreover, an increase of BMI by 1 unit was found to be associated with a 1.1–fold greater risk for developing SUI than POP.

Obesity appears to be a modifiable factor for remission of UI in women. Subak et al. [125] conducted a randomized controlled trial on 338 overweight and obese incontinent women. They reported that a moderate weight loss program reduced the frequency of incontinence episodes by approximately 50% and 7% of overweight women with frequent UI who became continent after a mean weight loss of 7.8 kg over a 6–month period after intervention. The following recommendations for preventing UI during pregnancy and the postpartum period involved maintaining normal weight before pregnancy (Grade B), and regaining pre–pregnancy weight postpartum (Grade B) [109]. In addition, the women with BMI ≤ 25 kg/m^2 at two years after delivery were a protective factor against UI (OR = 0.8, 95% CI = 0.77–0.98) [117].

Postpartum weight loss can decrease the risk for UI and promote the continence mechanism after delivery [112, 125]. Wesnes et al. [112] indicated that each kilogram of weight loss from delivery to 6 months postpartum among women who were incontinent during pregnancy decreases the relative risk for UI by 2.1% (relative risk 0.98, 95% confidence interval: 0.97, 0.99). Therefore, weight loss postpartum may be important to decreased incidence and increased remission of UI at 6 months postpartum and should, therefore, be addressed during continence promotion. According to Wing et al. [126], weight loss of 5–10% improves UI in obese and overweight women. It has been verified that weight loss improves the state of incontinence. Weight loss also leads to decreases in intravesical pressure and increases in valsalva leak point pressure [127].

Therefore, the risk for postpartum UI will decrease if a woman avoids being overweight or obese. This is an independent role for midwives who provide information and consultation for every woman to restore her pre–pregnancy weight [113]. Midwives can make a major contribution towards the prevention and rehabilitation of UI in women [113]. Interventions to prevent postpartum SUI in women should be implemented during both the antenatal and postpartum periods. The prevention of postpartum SUI should begin during pregnancy; pregnant women should be advised to modify behavior during pregnancy to control weight and thereby reduce their risk for postpartum SUI [124]. Midwives should implement the interventions for women during the postpartum period to help avoid weight retention. Individualized advice about eating and exercise habits to avoid weight retention after pregnancy may have a considerable impact on decreasing the risk for postpartum UI [113]. If possible, obese women should be offered nutritional consultation before pregnancy in order to reduce body weight [116].

5. Smoking

Smoking is also a contributing risk factor for SUI [128, 129]. Carbon monoxide in cigarettes impairs tissue oxygenation and results in muscle atrophy. The pelvic floor muscles are also affected. Chronic and frequent coughing exerting significant pressure on the pelvic floor muscles may lead to damaging innervation to the pelvic floor muscle and aggravate UI. Not only carbon monoxide, but also nicotine has a stimulating effect on the detrusor muscles. The chronic nicotinic detrusor muscle stimulation accompanied by increased intra–abdominal pressure contributes to urine leakage [130].

Hojberg et al. [59] reported pregnant women who smoke to be at a significantly higher risk for UI during pregnancy compared to non–smoking pregnant women (OR 1.4; 95% CI 1.1–1.9). Martins et al. [68] reported that 12.4% of Brazilian women smoke during pregnancy, and found a significant association between UI and smoking among incontinent pregnant women ($p = 0.010$). Similarly, Liang et al. [123] found 6.8% of pregnant women who reported smoking in pregnancy, a behavior associated with UUI, but found no association with SUI. Wesnes and Lose [109] recommended that women should be advised not to smoke before or during pregnancy in order to prevent UI during pregnancy and the postpartum period (Grade B).

6. Constipation

Women may experience constipation during the postpartum period. Constipation is defined as a functional bowel disorder characterized by pain and discomfort, straining, hard lumpy stools and a sense of incomplete bowel evacuation, which makes diagnosis both subjective and objective [131]. Constipation is a common condition affecting women during the postpartum period [132]. Bradley et al. [133] reported the prevalence of postpartum constipation to be estimated to be 24% at three months postpartum. Another study by Ponce et al. [134] reported a prevalence of constipation during the puerperium period as 41.8% by self–report. Evidence from studies suggests that a great number of women experience constipation up to three to six months postpartum. In some individuals, constipation may even persist to 12 months following delivery [135].

Pain or discomfort at the episiotomy site, the effects of pregnancy hormones such as progesterone and iron supplementation can increase the risk for postpartum constipation. Injury to the pelvic floor muscles or levator ani muscles during childbirth may lead to constipation during the postpartum period [136]. Other studies have found that forceps delivery, prolonged second stage of labor and higher child birth weight can result in anal sphincter injury resulting in postpartum constipation [137]. Hemorrhoids are also a common anorectal medical condition during pregnancy and the postpartum period causing painful defecation and swelling at the anus and resulting in constipation. Some other specific postpartum factors such as breastfeeding and obstetric events seem to affect bowel function during the postpartum period [133]. These changes may result in hard and dry stools potentially causing damage to the anal sphincter and pelvic floor muscles during defecation [131, 133].

Constipation may be associated as a risk for UI as the hard stool presses on the urethra, thereby affecting nerve innervation and blood flow to the urethral sphincter and potentially resulting in sphincteric deficiency [138]. In addition, constipation adds significant pressure to the bladder and urethra during defecation, which may also lead to UI. Amselem et al. [139] found constipation to be identified in 31% (19/61) of women with pelvic floor damage. In women without pelvic floor damage, constipation was present in 16% (83/535). These results indicate constipation to be as important as obstetric trauma in the development of PFM damage, which can cause postpartum UI. Zhu et al. [45] reported that women with a history of constipation were more likely to develop UI in late pregnancy (OR=1.218) and that difficult defecation was a risk factor for the development of UI from late pregnancy to 6 weeks postpartum (OR = 1.629).

In conclusion, many studies have found an association between constipation and postpartum UI. Therefore, prevention and treatment of constipation might significantly reduce the prevalence of UI during the postpartum period. Wesnes and Gunnar Lose [109] recommended that constipation should be avoided during pregnancy (evidence Grade B) and the postpartum period (evidence

Grade C) as a means of UI prevention for women during pregnancy and the postpartum period.

Turawa et al. [131] recommended a high-fiber diet and increased fluid intake to prevent constipation during the puerperium period. Pain–relief drugs and laxatives are common drugs for relieving constipation during the postpartum period [131]. Laxatives are grouped by function as follows: bulk-forming laxatives (such as bran, psyllium and methycellulose) that increase the weight and water content of stool to facilitate bowel movement; osmotic laxatives (such as lactulose and polyethylene glycol (PEG)) that add water to the colon to improve bowel movement; and stimulant laxatives (such as bisacodyl, castor oil and senna) that act by irritating the intestinal wall. Stool softeners lubricate stools to improve passage [131]. Although a high–fiber diet and increased fluid intake are encouraged to assist defecation during the puerperium period, pain–relief drugs and laxatives are common drugs of choice for alleviating constipation. However, the effectiveness and safety of laxatives in nursing mothers needs to be ascertained [131].

Unfortunately, the Cochrane review could not make explicit conclusions on interventions for treating postpartum constipation because the researchers found no studies for inclusion in this review [131].

7. Pre-Pregnancy and Antepartum Urinary Incontinence

Urinary incontinence starting during pregnancy is an important risk factor for UI after pregnancy [7, 89, 140–142] and later in life [29, 143]. New onset of UI during pregnancy could have an independent role and increase the risk for postpartum SUI [67, 84]. Urine leakage prior the current pregnancy or in previous pregnancies could be a sign of poor quality of the connective tissue of the pelvic floor muscle [144] and may reduce fascia tensile strength during pregnancy more than in previously continent women [145]. The weakness of the pelvic floor muscle resulting in the loss of the supportive mechanism of the urethra and bladder neck further contributes to the risk for SUI [144]. The mean value of the pelvic floor contraction strength at 6 months after delivery is also significantly lower among the incontinent women [67].

Pre–pregnancy SUI is also indicated as a risk factor for developing UI during pregnancy and during the postpartum period. Published findings have further indicated that pregnancy UI is an independent risk factor for incontinence during the postpartum period [89, 105, 140]. Hvidman et al. [34] reported that previously incontinent pregnant women had significantly higher risk for SUI during pregnancy than previously continent pregnant women (OR 10.6). Van Brummen et al. [141] stated that new onset of SUI during pregnancy was the most effective factor in the development of SUI after childbirth. Eason et al. [105] indicated that UI during pregnancy increased the risk for presenting symptoms of UI at 3 months after delivery by a factor of 1.9. Foldspang et al. [142] monitored 1,232 women from 12 to 120 months postpartum. Of the 16% who had antenatal UI, 67% reported postpartum UI compared with only 19% of those without antenatal UI. According to the study of Stainton et al. [146], women who experience urine leakage prior to pregnancy are at risk for and contribute to postpartum UI (P = 0.02). These findings are supported by Brown et al. [9] who examined the association between pre–pregnancy UI and pregnancy UI in 1,507 nulliparous women. According to the findings, the women who developed UI during pregnancy had a substantially higher likelihood of incontinence following childbirth compared with those who were continent during pregnancy. According to the findings, the strongest predictor for incidence of UI during pregnancy was occasional pre–pregnancy urine leakage (AdjOR 3.6, 95% CI 2.8–4.7).

Urinary incontinence before the last trimester of pregnancy has also been found to be strongly associated with UI during the early postpartum period. Pizzoferrato et al. [147] found UI during pregnancy to be a strong risk factor for UI at 1 year postpartum (OR 6.27 [95% CI 2.70–14.6]). Similar to the findings of Hantoushzadeh's study [98] in women with pre-pregnancy history of SUI, primiparous women who had experienced SUI before pregnancy and complained of SUI at 1 year postpartum more frequently [73%] compared to their control group [12.6%, P < 0.001, RR = 5.75]. Svare et al. [116] reported that SUI or MUI at 1 year after the first vaginal delivery was strongly associated with UI during pregnancy [adjOR 4.7, 95 %CI 2.9–7.7]. The indication is that some women may develop more pronounced pelvic floor dysfunction and, therefore, experience UI during their first pregnancy. This seems to be a strong risk factor for UI at 1 year after delivery. Brown et al. [75] found women experiencing UI during the index pregnancy to have the highest likelihood for postpartum incontinence (adjusted OR 3.3). Diez–Itza et al. [67] conducted a longitudinal study in 352 primigravid women to investigate the risk factors involved in SUI at 1 year after first delivery. According to the findings, the only factor independently associated with SUI after delivery was the development of SUI during pregnancy (OR, 5.79; 95% CI, 2.79–12.00). Therefore, the conclusion was drawn that new onset of SUI during pregnancy is an independent risk factor for SUI during the postpartum period.

Urinary incontinence during the first pregnancy increases the long-term risk for UI and decreases the chance of remission between 4 and 12 years [75]. Barbosa et al. [148] found women with UI during pregnancy to be more likely to describe UI symptoms 2 years after delivery (OR = 8.6, 95% CI = 3.0–24.3). Liang et al. [149] found primiparous women who had UI during their first pregnancy to be more likely to develop UI at 5 years postpartum than women who had no UI during their first pregnancy.

Antenatal UI increases the risk for postpartum UI, which in turn increases the risk for long–term persistent UI after delivery [84]. In a cohort study, Wesnes et al. [89] conducted a survey of 12,679 primigravid women who were continent before pregnancy to investigate the prevalence of UI at 6 months postpartum in primiparous women. According to the findings, urinary incontinence was reported by 31% of the women at 6 months after delivery. Furthermore, women who experienced UI at Week 30 of pregnancy were at statistically significant risk for persistent UI at 6 months postpartum with an adjusted RR of 2.3 (adjusted RR 2.3, 95% CI 2.2–2.4) compared with women who were continent at Week 30. The majority of women reporting persistent UI at 4–18 months after delivery also experience symptoms during pregnancy. Gartland et al. [150] found women who reported UI before pregnancy to have a seven–fold increase in odds of persistent UI between 4 and 18 months postpartum compared with women who were continent during pregnancy (aOR 7.4, 95% CI 5.1–10.7).

8. Women with Gestational Diabetes Mellitus (GDM) or a History of Gestational Diabetes Mellitus (hGDM)

Gestational diabetes mellitus (GDM) is a condition involving carbohydrate intolerance resulting from inadequate insulin supply first recognized or developed during pregnancy with varying perinatal morbidity and mortality rates [151]. Few studies have reported pregnant women with GDM to have a high prevalence of UI [152, 153]. Although the associations between diabetes mellitus and urinary incontinence as well as the associations between pregnancy and UI are well–established, the associations between GDM and UI have rarely been investigated [154].

In non–pregnant women, women with diabetes mellitus are 50–200% more likely to experience UI compared with women with normal glucose levels [154]. The factors potentially contributing to UI in diabetes mellitus include microvascular damage, insulin injection and disease duration [155,

156]. Furthermore, diabetic bladder dysfunction has been linked to the etiologies of UI. The early phase of diabetic bladder dysfunction presents as a storage problem such as urgency and urge incontinence, whereas the late phase manifests as voiding problems leading to high residual urine and overflow incontinence [157].

In pregnant women, women who have GDM also have a high prevalence of UI due to higher BMI, excess weight, obesity and macrosomia of infants [152,153]. However, the exact mechanism remains unclear and excess weight gain during pregnancy may exert pressure on the pelvic floor muscle, which increases pressure on the bladder and urethral mobility, thereby leading to UI [158].

At present, only one relevant report has found a positive relationship between GDM and SUI during the postpartum period. In a longitudinal cohort study, Chuang et al. [154] conducted a survey of 6,653 pregnant women with GDM to determine whether or not GDM is an independent risk factor for SUI postpartum. According to the findings, pregnant women with GDM are more likely to develop all three types of UI and have poor QoL during the postpartum period. Also according to the findings, pregnant women with GDM tend to exhibit more severe SUI symptoms for up 2 years postpartum compared than women without GDM (OR 1.97, 95% CI 1.56–2.51), thereby indicating that the impact of GDM on postpartum genitourinary function is relatively prolonged in these women. The aforementioned finding contradicts the common belief that the effects of GDM usually vanish soon after delivery. Therefore, the researchers concluded that GDM was found to be an independent risk factor for UI postpartum that is significantly associated with impact on QOL [154].

Furthermore, a history of gestational diabetes mellitus (hGDM) has also been found to have a positive association with SUI during the postpartum period. In a cross–sectional survey, Kim et al. [159] examined the prevalence of SUI among women with hGDM by surveying 228 women with hGDM for 5 years after delivery and finding 49% of the women with hGDM to report weekly or more frequent incontinence during pregnancy, while 50% of the women reported postpartum SUI. Therefore, a high prevalence of obesity may have contributed to the high prevalence of SUI during pregnancy and after delivery among the participants. The afornentioned study found obesity in 42% of women during pregnancy and 46% after delivery. However, there was no clear association between BMI and SUI. Thus, the researchers concluded that SUI was common among women with hGDM.

DISCUSSION AND CONCLUSION

With regard to the aforementioned findings, the prevalence of UI during the postpartum period ranged from 6.9% [10] to 47.0% [11], which is lower when compared with the prevalence during the third trimester of pregnancy. However, the remission rate for UI at three months after childbirth as high as 86.4% [12]. This means that not all postpartum women develop postpartum UI. Therefore, approximately more than half (53%) of these women will not develop UI following childbirth.

It is well known that UI during pregnancy and the postpartum period is associated with inadequate pelvic floor muscle strength. Women who developed UI during pregnancy have a substantially increased risk for UI following childbirth compared with those who are continent during pregnancy. Therefore, any factors causing weakening of pelvic floor muscle strength are likely to be causal factors for UI during pregnancy and the postpartum period. Several factors may decrease the strength of pelvic floor muscles in addition to pregnancy itself [21].

Based on the aforementioned findings, it can be concluded that the main risk factors contributing to the development of postpartum UI include the following 8 risk factors: 1) maternal age, 2) parity, 3) mode of delivery, 4) obesity, 5) smoking, 6) constipation, 7) pre-pregnancy UI or antepartum UI, and 8) gestational diabetes mellitus (GDM) or history of GDM. These findings concur with a literature review by Cerruto et al. [12], which found the main risk factors for postpartum UI to be maternal age, parity, maternal overweight and UI during pregnancy. In 2014, Sangsawang [21] published the results of a literature review, concluding that no associations were found among aforementioned risk factors. This means that each risk factor is independent and will independently result in postpartum UI. Therefore, pregnant or postpartum women do not need to have all of the risk factors in order to develop UI after delivery. Pregnant women and postpartum mothers may have only one or a combination of multiple risk factors to cause UI and various risk factors will result in inadaquate pelvic floor muscle strength with the possibility of developing UI.

According from the published literature review by Sangsawang [21], the mechanisms involved in developing SUI during pregnancy are included in the following 3 domains: 1) increased intra–abdominal pressure; 2) direct increased pressure on the bladder, urethra and pelvic floor muscle and 3) impaired blood flow, oxygen transportation and innervation to the bladder, urethra and pelvic floor muscles .The aforementioned factors have the effect of weakening the pelvic floor muscles, the major support of the continence mechanism, and lead to pelvic floor and urethral dysfunction with loss of urethral closure pressure [21]. Therefore, the postpartum UI has risk factors that can be attributed to the weakening of the pelvic floor muscles during the postpartum period, which is similar to UI during pregnancy.

For example, the first domain, increased intra–abdominal pressure, may include constipation and smoking. The secondary domain, increased pressure to the bladder, urethra and pelvic floor muscle may include parity, mode of delivery, obesity and history of GDM. The final domain, impaired blood flow, oxygen transportation and innervation to the bladder, urethra and pelvic floor muscle may include mode of delivery and obesity.

In addition, parity, mode of delivery, obesity, smoking, and constipation are independent risk factors for UI both during pregnancy and after childbirth. These factors can be avoided and prevented with behavioral modification during pregnancy and the postpartum period. Effective means of preventing postpartum UI are aimed at strengthening the pelvic floor muscles and avoiding the risks factors for weakening pelvic floor muscle strength.

To decrease the risk for postpartum UI, pregnant women might perform pelvic floor muscle exercises (PFME) which might help prevent postpartum UI. Therefore, women should be advised to perform PFME during pregnancy and the postpartum period. Furthermore, cesarean section seems to be followed by less postpartum UI than vaginal delivery or instrumental vaginal delivery. Therefore, elective cesarean section in women also has a protective effect and lowers the risk for developing postpartum UI. Moreover, postpartum weight loss by advice about eating and exercise habits to avoid weight retention after delivery can also decrease the risk for UI and regain the continence mechanism at six months postpartum. In addition, all women should be advised not to smoke before or during pregnancy and constipation should be avoided during pregnancy to prevent UI during pregnancy and the postpartum period. A high–fiber diet and increased fluid intake can prevent constipation during the postpartum period.

Nevertheless, non–modifiable, genetic and obstetric risk factors such as maternal age, pre–pregnancy UI and GDM have an important role in UI postpartum development. Factors such as parity, mode of delivery, obesity, smoking and constipation are modifiable risk factors. Avoiding modifiable risk factors might reduce the risk for development of UI in postpartum women. Moreover, the prevention of UI during pregnancy may also reduce the incidence of postpartum UI after delivery and persistent postpartum UI in later years after childbirth [21].

REFERENCES

[1] Haylen, B. T., de Ridder, D., Freeman, R. M., et al. (2010). An International Urogyneco-logical Association (IUGA)/International Continence Society (ICS) joint report on the terminology for female pelvic floor dysfunction. *Int Urogynecol J*, 21(1), 5–26.

[2] Ege, E., Akin, B., Altuntuğ, K., Benli, S., and Arioz, A. (2008). Prevalence of urinary incontinence in the 12-month postpartum period and related risk factors in Turkey. *Urol Int*, 80(4), 355-61.

[3] Hermansen, I. L., O'Connell, B. O., and Gaskin, C. J. (2010). Women's explanations for urinary incontinence, their management strategies, and their quality of life during the postpartum period. *Wound Ostomy Continence Nurs*, 37(2), 187-92.

[4] Mascarenhas, T., Coelho, R., Oliveira, M., and Patricio, B. (2003). Impact of urinary incontinence on quality of life during pregnancy and after childbirth. Paper presented at the 33rd annual meeting of the International Continence Society, Florence, Italy, 5th - 9th October, 2003.

[5] Sword, W., Landy, C. K., Thabane, L., et al. (2011). Is mode of delivery associated with postpartum depression at 6 weeks: a prospective cohort study. *Br J Obstet Gynaecol*, 118(8), 966-77.

[6] Goyeneche. L., Uranga, S., Salgueiro, M. D., Lekuona, A., Sarasqueta, C., and Diez Itza, I .(2013). Influence of urinary incontinence on postpartum depression and anxiety. Paper presented at the 43rd annual meeting of the International Continence Society, Barcelona, Spain, 26th - 30th August, 2013.

[7] Schytt, E., Lindmark, G., and Waldenstrom, U. (2004). Symptoms of stress incontinence 1 year after childbirth: prevalence and predictors in a national Swedish sample. *Acta Obstet Gynecol Scand*, 83, 928–936.

[8] Martínez Franco, E., Parés, D., Lorente Colomé, N., Méndez Paredes, J. R., and Amat Tardiu, L. (2014). Urinary incontinence during pregnancy. Is there a difference between first and third trimester? *Eur J Obstet Gynecol Reprod Biol*, 182, 86-90.

[9] Brown, S. J., Donath, S., MacArthur, C., McDonald, E. A., and Krastev, A. H. (2010). Urinary incontinence in nulliparous women before and during pregnancy: prevalence, incidence, and associated risk factors. *Int Urogynecol J*, 21(2), 193-202.

[10] Martin-Martin, S., Pascual-Fernandez, A., Alvarez-Colomo, C., Calvo-Gonzalez, R., Muñoz-Moreno, M., and Cortiñas-Gonzalez, J. R. (2014). Urinary incontinence during pregnancy and postpartum. Associated risk

factors and influence of pelvic floor exercises. *Arch Esp Urol,* 67(4), 323-30.

[11] Brown, S., Gartland, D., Perlen, S., McDonald, E., and MacArthur, C. (2015). Consultation about urinary and faecal incontinence in the year after childbirth: a cohort study. *Br J Obstet Gynaecol*, 122(7), 954-62.

[12] Cerruto, M. A., D'Elia, C., Aloisi, A., Fabrello, M., and Artibani, W. (2013). Prevalence, incidence and obstetric factors' impact on female urinary incontinence in Europe: a systematic review. *Urol Int*, 90(1), 1-9.

[13] Fritel, X., Ringa, V., Quiboeuf, E., and Fauconnier, A. (2012). Female urinary incontinence, from pregnancy to menopause: a review of epidemiological and pathophysiological findings. *Acta Obstet Gynecol Scand*, 91, 901–10.

[14] Dietz, H. P., Eldridge, A., Grace, M., and Clarke, B. (2012). Does pregnancy affect pelvic organ mobility? *Aust N Z J Obstet Gynaecol*, 44, 517-20.

[15] King, J. K., and Freeman, R.M. (1998). Is antenatal bladder neck mobility a risk factor for postpartum stress incontinence? *Br J Obstet Gynaecol*, 105, 1300-7.

[16] Toozs-Hobson, P., Balmforth, J., Cardozo, L., Khullar, V., and Athanasiou, S. (2008). The effect of mode of delivery on pelvic floor functional anatomy. *Int Urogynecol J Pelvic Floor Dysfunct*,19, 407–16.

[17] Van Geelen, J. M, Lemmens, W. A. J. G., Eskes, T. K. A. B., and Martin, C. B. (1982). The urethral pressure profile in pregnancy and after delivery in healthy nulliparous women. *Am J Obstet Gynecol*, 114, 636-49.

[18] DeLancey, J. O. L. (2010). Why do women have stress urinary incontinence? *Neurourol Urodyn*, 29, S13-17.

[19] FitzGerald, M. P, and Graziano, S. (2007). Anatomic and functional changes of the lower urinary tract during pregnancy. *Urol Clin North Am*, 34, 7–12.

[20] McKinnie, V., Swift, S. E., Wang, W., et al. (2005). The effect of pregnancy and mode of delivery on the prevalence of urinary and fecal incontinence. *Am J Obstet Gynecol*,193, 512–8.

[21] Sangsawang, B. (2014). Risk factors for the development of stress urinary incontinence during pregnancy in primigravidae: a review of literatures. *Eur J Obstet Gynecol Reprod Biol*, 178, 27–34.

[22] Viktrup, L. (2002). The risk of urinary tract symptom five years after the first delivery. *Neurourol Urodyn*, 21(1), 2–29.

[23] Sangsawang, B., and Sangsawang, N. (2013). Stress urinary incontinence in pregnant women: a review of prevalence, pathophysiology, and treatment. *Int Urogynecol J*, 24(6),901-912.

[24] Pregazzi, R., Sartore, A., Troiano, L., et al. (2002). Postpartum urinary symptoms: prevalence and risk factors. *Eur J Obstet Gynecol Reprod Biol*, 103(2), 179-82.

[25] Quiboeuf, E., Saurel-Cubizolles, M. J., Fritel, X., and EDEN Mother-Child Cohort Study Group. (2016). Trends in urinary incontinence in women between 4 and 24 months postpartum in the EDEN cohort. *Br J Obstet Gynaecol*, 123(7), 1222-8.

[26] Chaliha, C., Kalia,V., Stanton, S. L., Monga, A., and Sultan, A.H. (1999). Antenatal prediction of postpartum urinary and fecal incontinence. *Obst Gynaecol*, 94, 689–94.

[27] Handa, V. L., Harris, T. A., and Ostergard, D. R. (1996). Protecting the pelvic floor: obstetric management to prevent incontinence and pelvic organ prolapse. *Obstet Gynecol*, 88, 470–8.

[28] Connolly, A. M., and Thorp Jr, J. M. (1999). Childbirth-related perineal trauma: clinical significance and prevention. *Clin Obstet Gynecol*, 42(4), 820–35.

[29] Viktrup, L., Rortveit, G., and Lose, G. (2006). Risk of stress urinary incontinence twelve years after the first pregnancy and delivery. *Obstet Gynecol*, 108(2), 248–254.

[30] Thom, D. H., and Rortveit, G. (2010). Prevalence of postpartum urinary incontinence: a systematic review. *Acta Obstet Gynecol Scand*, 89(12),1511–1522.

[31] Viktrup L, Lose G, Rolf M, and Barfoed, K. (1993). The frequency of urinary symptoms during pregnancy and puerperium in the primipara. *Int Urogynecol J*, 4(1), 27–30.

[32] Pizzoferrato, A.C., Fauconnier, A., Quiboeuf, E., Morel, K., Schaal, J. P., and Fritel, X. (2014). Urinary incontinence 4 and 12 years after first delivery: risk factors associated with prevalence, incidence, remission, and persistence in a cohort of 236 women. *Neurourol Urodyn*, 33(8), 1229-34.

[33] Arrue, M., Ibañez, L., Paredes, J., et al. (2010). Stress urinary incontinence six months after first vaginal delivery. *Eur J Obstet Gynecol Reprod Biol*, 150(2), 210–214.

[34] Hvidman, L., Foldspang, A., Mommsen, S., and Bugge Nielsen, J. (2002). Correlates of urinary incontinence in pregnancy. *Int Urogynecol J Pelvic Floor Dysfunct*, 13(5), 278–283.

[35] Serati, M., Salvatore, S., Khullar, V., et al. (2008). Prospective study to assess risk factors for pelvic floor dysfunction after delivery. *Acta Obstet Gynecol Scand*, 87(3), 313–318.

[36] Thomason, A. D., Miller, J. M., and Delancey, J. O. (2007). Urinary incontinence symptoms during and after pregnancy in continent and incontinent primiparas. *Int Urogynecol J Pelvic Floor Dysfunct*, 18(2), 147–151.

[37] Nygaard, I., Barber, M. D., Burgio, K. L., et al. (2008). Prevalence of symptomatic pelvic floor disorders in US women. *JAMA*, 300(11), 1311–6.

[38] Tinelli, A., Malvasi, A., Rahimi, S., et al. (2010). Age-related pelvic floor modifications and prolapse risk factors in postmenopausal women. *Menopause: J N Am Menopause Soc,*17(1), 204–12.

[39] Swift, S., Woodman, P., O'Boyle, A., et al. (2005). Pelvic Organ Support Study (POSST): the distribution, clinical definition, and epidemiologic condition of pelvic organ support defects. *Am J Obstet Gynaecol*, 192(3),795–806.

[40] Patel, D. A., Xu, X., Thomason, A. D., Ransom, S. B., Ivy, J. S., and DeLancey, J. O. L. (2006). Childbirth and pelvic floor dysfunction: an epidemiologic approach to the assessment of prevention opportunities at delivery. *Am J Obstet Gynaecol*, 195(1), 23–8.

[41] Gyhagen, M., Bullarbo, M., Nielsen, T. F., and Milsom, I. (2012). Prevalence and risk factors for pelvic organ prolapse 20 years after childbirth: a national cohort study in singleton primiparae after vaginal or caesarean delivery. *Br J Obstet Gynaecol*, 120(2), 152–60.

[42] Wilson, D., Dornan, J., Milsom, I., and Freeman, R. (2014). UR-CHOICE: can we provide mothers-to-be with information about the risk of future pelvic floor dysfunction? *Int Urogynecol J*, 25,1449–52.

[43] Wesnes, S. L., Rortveit, G., Bø, K., and Hunskaar, S. (2007). Urinary incontinence during pregnancy. *Obstet Gynecol*, 109(4), 922-928.

[44] Obioha, K. C., Ugwu, E. O., Obi, S. N., Dim, C. C., and Oguanuo, T. C. (2015). Prevalence and predictors of urinary/anal incontinence after vaginal delivery: prospective study of Nigerian women. *Int Urogynecol J*, 26,1347–1354.

[45] Zhu, L., Li, L., Lang, J. H., and Xu, T. (2012). Prevalence and risk factors for peri and postpartum urinary incontinence in primiparous women in China: a prospective longitudinal study. *Int Urogynecol J*, 23(5), 563-572.

[46] MacArthur, C., Glazener, C., DonWilson, P., Lancashire, R., Herbison, G., and Grant, A. (2006). Persistent urinary incontinence and delivery mode history: a six-year longitudinal study. *Br J Obstet Gynaecol*, 113, 218–224.

[47] Glazener, C. M., Herbison, G. P., MacArthur, C., et al. (2006). New postnatal urinary incon-tinence: obstetric and other risk factors in primiparae. *Br J Obstet Gynaecol*, 113(2), 208-217.

[48] Allahdin, S. and Kambhampati, L. (2012). Stress urinary incontinence in continent primigravidas. *J Obstet Gynaecol*, 32(1), 2-5.

[49] Groutz, A., Helpman, L., Gold, R., Pauzner, D., Lessing, J. B., and Gordon, D. (2007). First vaginal delivery at an older age: Does it carry an extra risk for the development of stress urinary incontinence? *Neurourol Urodyn*, 26(6), 779-782.

[50] Dietz, H. P. and Wilson, P. D. (2005). Childbirth and pelvic floor trauma. *Best Pract Res Clin Obstet Gynaecol*, 19, 913-924.

[51] Rud, T. (1980). Urethral pressure profile in continent women from childhood to old age. *Acta Obstet Gynecol Scand*, 59, 331-335.

[52] Pandit, M., DeLancey, J. O., Ashton-Miller, J. A., Iyengar, J., Blaivas, M., and Perucchini, D. (2000). Quantification of intramuscular nerves within the female striated urogenital sphincter muscle. *Obstet Gynecol*, 95, 797-800.

[53] Perucchini, D., DeLancey, J. O., Ashton-Miller, J. A., Peschers, U., and Kataria, T. (2002). Age effects on urethral striated muscle. I. Changes in number and diameter of striated muscle fibers in the ventral urethra. *Am J Obstet Gynecol*, 186, 351-355.

[54] Iyoke, C.A., Ezugwu, F.O., and Onal, H. E. (2010). Prevalence and correlates of maternal morbidity in Enugu, South-East Nigeria. *Afr J Reprod Health*, 14,121–129.

[55] Ezegwui, H. U., Ikeakor, L. C., and Egbuji, C. (2011). Fetal macrosomia: obstetric outcome of 311 cases inUNTH, Enugu, Nigeria. *Niger J Clin Pract*, 14, 332–336.

[56] Hijaz, A., Sadeghi, Z., Byrne, L., Hou, J. C., and Daneshgari, F. (2012). Advanced maternal age as a risk factor for stress urinary incontinence: a review of the literature. *Int Urogynecol J*, 23, 395-401.

[57] Trowbridge, E. R., Wei, J. T., Fenner, D. E., Ashton-Miller, J. A., and Delancey, J. O. (2007). Effects of aging on lower urinary tract and pelvic floor function in nulliparous women. *Obstet Gynecol*, 109(3), 715-720.

[58] Ebbesen, M. H., Hunskaar, S., Rortveit, G., et al. (2013). Prevalence, incidence and remission of urinary incontinence in women: longitudinal

data from the Norwegian HUNT study (EPINCONT). *BMC Urology*, 13, 27.

[59] Hojberg, K. E., Salvig, J. D., Winslow, N. A., Lose, G., and Secher, N. J. (1999). Urinary incontinence: prevalence and risk factors at 16 weeks of gestation. *Br J Obstet Gynaecol*, 106, 842-850.

[60] Lewicky-Gaupp, C., Cao, D. C. and Culbertson, S. (2008). Urinary and anal incontinence in African American teenaged gravidas during pregnancy and the puerperium. *J Pediatr Adolesc Gynecol*, 21(1), 21-26.

[61] Rodríguez-Mias, N. L., Martínez-Franco, E., Aguado, J., Sánchez., E, and Amat-Tardiu, L. (2015). Pelvic organ prolapse and stress urinary incontinence, do they share the same risk factors? *Eur J Obstet Gynecol Reprod Biol*, 190, 52–57.

[62] Rortveit, G., Hannestad, Y. S., Daltveit, A. K., and Hunskaar, S. (2001). Ageand type-dependent effects of parity on urinary incontinence: the Norwegian EPICONT study. *Obstet Gynecol*, 98, 1004–1010.

[63] Assassa, R., Dallosso, H., Perry, S., et al. (2000). The association between obstetric factors and incontinence: a community survey. *Br J Obstet Gynaecol*, 107, 822.

[64] Goldberg, R., Kwon, C., Gandhi, S., Atkuru, L., Sornsen, M., and Sand, P. (2003). Urinary incontinence among mothers of multiples: the protective effect of cesarean delivery. *Am J Obstet Gynecol*, 188, 1447–1450.

[65] Wilson, P., and Herbison, G. (2003). A randomized controlled trial of pelvic floor muscle exercises to treat postnatal urinary incontinence. *Int Urogynecol J Pelvic Floor Dysfunct*, 9, 257–264.

[66] Özdemır, Ö. Ç., Bakar, Y., Özengın, N., and Duran, B. (2015). The effect of parity on pelvic floor muscle strength and quality of life in women with urinary incontinence: a cross sectional study. *J Phys Ther Sci*, 27, 2133–2137.

[67] Diez-Itza, I., Arrue, M., Ibañez, L., Murgiondo, A., Paredes, J., and Sarasqueta, C. (2010). Factors involved in stress urinary incontinence 1 year after first delivery. *Int Urogynecol J*, 21, 439–445.

[68] Martins, G., Soler, Z. A., Cordeiro, J. A., Amaro, J. L., and Moore, K. N. (2010). Prevalence and risk factors for urinary incontinence in healthy pregnant Brazilian women. *Int Urogynecol J*, 21(10), 1271-1277.

[69] Meyer, S., Schreyer, A., Grandi, P., and Hohlfeld, P. (1998). The effect of birth on urinary incontinence mechanisms and other pelvic-floor characteristics. *Obstet Gynecol*, 92(4), 613-618.

[70] Marshall, K., Thompson, K. A., Walsh, D. M., and Baxter, G. D. (1998). Incidence of urinary incontinence and constipation during pregnancy and postpartum: survey of current findings at the Rotunda Lying-in Hospital. *Br J Obstet Gynaecol*, 105, 400-402.

[71] Riesco, M. L., Caroci, A.S., de Oliveira, S.M., et al. (2010). Perineal muscle strength during pregnancy and postpartum: the correlation between perineo-metry and digital vaginal palpation. *Rev Lat Am Enfermagem*, 18, 1138–1144.

[72] Payne, C.K. (2008). Epidemiology, pathophysiology, and evaluation of urinary incontinence and overactive bladder. *Urology*, 51, 3-10.

[73] Zahariou, A.G., Karamouti, M. V., and Papaioannou, P.D. (2008). Pelvic floor muscle training improves sexual function of women with stress urinary incontinence. *Int Urogynecol J Pelvic Floor Dysfunct*, 3, 401-406.

[74] Shek, K. L., Kruger, J., and Dietz, H. P. (2012). The effect of pregnancy on hiatal dimensions and urethral mobility: an observational study. *Int Urogynecol J*, 23, 1561-7.

[75] Brown, S., Gartland, D., Donath, S., and MacArthur, C. (2011). Effects of prolonged second stage, method of birth, timing of caesarean section and other obstetric risk factors on postnatal urinary incontinence: an Australian nulliparous cohort study. *Br J Obstet Gynaecol*, 118, 991–1000.

[76] Meyer, S., Bachelard, O. and De Grandi, P. (1998). Do bladder neck mobility and urethral sphincter function differ during pregnancy compared with during the non-pregnant state? *Int Urogynecol J Pelvic Floor Dysfunct*, 9(6), 397-404.

[77] Zhu, L., Bian, X. M., Long, Y., and Lang, J. H. (2008). Role of different childbirth strategies on pelvic organ prolapse and stress urinary incontinence: a prospective study. *Chin Med J*, 121(3), 213-215.

[78] Chaliha, C. (2009). Postpartum pelvic floor trauma. *Curr Opin Obstet Gynecol*, 21(6), 474-479.

[79] Herbruck, L. F. (2008). The impact of childbirth on the pelvic floor. *Urol Nurs*, 28(3),173-184.

[80] Rørtveit, G., and Hannestad, Y. S. (2014). Association between mode of delivery and pelvic floor dysfunction. *Tidsskr Nor Laegeforen*, 134(19), 1848-52.

[81] Tunn, R., Goldammer, K., Neymeyer, J., Gauruder-Burmester, A., Hamm, B., and Beyersdorff, D. (2006). MRI morphology of the levator

ani muscle, endopelvic fascia, and urethra in women with stress urinary incontinence. *Eur J Obstet Gynecol Reprod Biol*, 126(2), 239-245.

[82] Rogers, R. G., Leeman, L. M., Borders, N., et al. (2014). Contribution of the second stage of labour to pelvic floor dysfunction: a prospective cohort comparison of nulliparous women. *Br J Obstet Gynaecol*, 121, 1145–1154.

[83] Peschers, U. M, Schaer, G.N., DeLancey, J. O., et al. (1997). Levator ani function before and after childbirth. *Br J Obstet Gynaecol*, 104, 1004–1008.

[84] Nygaard, I. (2006). Urinary Incontinence: Is Cesarean Delivery Protective? *Semin Perinatol*, 30, 267-271.

[85] Torrisi, G., Minini, G., Bernasconi, F., et al. (2012). A prospective study of pelvic floor dysfunctions related to delivery. *Eur J Obstet Gynecol Reprod Biol*, 160(1), 110-115.

[86] Leijonhufvud, A., Lundholm, C., Cnattingius, S., Granath, F., Andolf, E., and Altman, D. (2011). Risks of stress urinary incontinence and pelvic organ prolapse surgery in relation to mode of childbirth. *Am J Obstet Gynecol*, 204(1), 70. 1-7.

[87] Farrell S, Allen, V., and Baskett, T. (2001). Partuition and urinary incontinence in primiparas. *J Obstet Gynecol*, 97, 350- 356.

[88] Gyhagen, M., Bullarbo, M., Nielsen, T. F., and Milsom, I. (2013). A comparison of the long-term consequences of vaginal delivery versus caesarean section on the prevalence, severity and bothersomeness of urinary incontinence subtypes: a national cohort study in primiparous women. *Br J Obstet Gynaecol*, 120, 1548–1555.

[89] Wesnes, S. L., Hunskaar, S., Bo, K., and Rortveit, G. (2009). The effect of urinary incontinence status during pregnancy and delivery mode on incontinence postpartum. A cohort study. *Br J Obstet Gynaecol*, 116(5), 700-707.

[90] Arya, L. A., Jackson, N. D., Myers, D. L., and Verma, A. (2001). Risk of new-onset urinary incontinence after forceps and vacuum delivery in primiparous women. *Am J Obstet Gynecol*, 185(6), 1318-1324.

[91] Van Kessel, K., Reed, S., Newton, K., Meier, A., and Lentz, G. (2001). The second stage of labor and stress urinary incontinence. *Am J Obstet Gynecol*, 184(7),1571-1575.

[92] Yang, X., Zhang, H. X., Yu, H. Y., Gao, X. L., Yang, H. X., and Dong, Y. (2010). The prevalence of fecal incontinence and urinary incontinence in primiparous postpartum Chinese women. *Eur J Obstet Gynecol Reprod Biol*, 152(2), 214-217.

[93] Li, H., Wu, R.F., Qi, F., et al. (2015). Postpartum pelvic floor function performance after two different modes of delivery. *Genet Mol Res*, 14 (2), 2994-3001.

[94] Rortveit, G., Daltveit, A. K., Hannestad, Y. S., Hunskaar, S., and Norwegian EPINCONT Study. (2003). Urinary incontinence after vaginal delivery orcesarean section. *N Engl J Med*, 348, 900–7.

[95] Handa, V. L., Blomquist, J. L., McDermott, K. C., Friedman, S., and Munoz, A. (2012). Pelvic floor disorders after vaginal birth: effect of episiotomy, perineal laceration, and operative birth. *Obstet Gynecol*, 119(2 Pt 1), 233–9.

[96] Barber, E. L., Lundsberg, L.S., Belanger, K., Pettker, C. M., Funai, E. F., and Illuzzi, J. L. (2011). Indications contributing to the increasing caesarean delivery rate. *Obstet Gynecol*, 118, 29–38.

[97] Wax, J. R., Cartin, A., Pinette, M. G., and Blackstone, J. (2005). Patient choice caesarean– the Maine experience. *Birth*, 32, 203–6.

[98] Hantoushzadeh, S., Javadian, P., Shariat, M., Salmanian, B., Ghazizadeh, S., and Aghssa, M. (2011). Stress urinary incontinence: pre-pregnancy history and effects of mode of delivery on its postpartum persistency. *Int Urogynecol J*, 22(6), 651-655.

[99] Panayi, D. C. and Khullar, V. (2009). Urogynaecological problems in pregnancy and postpartum sequelae. *Curr Opin Obstet Gynecol*, 21(1), 97-100.

[100] Eftekhar, T., Hajibaratali, B., Ramezanzadeh, F., and Shariat, M. (2006). Postpartum evaluation of stress urinary incontinence among primiparas. *Int J Gynaecol Obstet*, 94(2), 114-118.

[101] Boyles, S. H., Li, H., Mori, T., Osterweil, P., and Guise, J. M. (2009). Effect of mode of delivery on the incidence of urinary incontinence in primiparous women. *Obstet Gynecol*, 113(1), 134-141.

[102] Mason, L., Glenn, S., Walton, I., et al. (1989). The prevalence of stress incontinence during pregnancy and following delivery. *Midwifery*,15, 120-128.

[103] Goldberg, R. P., Abramov, Y., Botros, S., et al. (2005). Delivery mode is a major environmental determinant of stress urinary incontinence: results of the Evanston-Northwestern Twin Sisters Study. *Am J Obstet Gynecol*, 193(6), 2149-2153.

[104] Chaliha, C, Khullar, V., Stanton, S. L., et al. (2002). Urinary symptoms in pregnancy: are they useful for diagnosis? *Br J Obstet Gynaecol*, 109, 1181-1183.

[105] Eason, E., Labrecque, M., Marcoux, S., et al. (2004). Effects of carrying a pregnancy and of method of delivery on urinary incontinence: a prospective cohort study. *BMC Pregnancy and Childbirth*, 4, 4.

[106] Groutz, A., Rimon, E., Peled, S., et al. (2004). Cesarean section: does it really prevent the development of postpartum stress urinary incontinence? A prospective study of 363 women one year after their first delivery. *Neurourol Urodyn*, 23, 2-6.

[107] Altman, D., Ekström, A., Forsgren, C., Nordenstam, J., and Zetterström, J. (2007). Symptoms of anal and urinary incontinence following cesarean section or spontaneous vaginal delivery. *Am J Obstet Gynecol*, 197(5), 512.1-7.

[108] Chou, P. L., Chen, F. P. and Teng, L. F. (2005). Factors associated with urinary stress incontinence in primiparas. *Taiwan J Obstet Gynecol*, 44, 42-47.

[109] Wesnes, S. L. and Lose, G. (2013). Preventing urinary incontinence during pregnancy and postpartum: a review. *Int Urogynecol J*, 24, 889–899.

[110] Wilson, P. D., Herbison, R. M. and Herbison, G. P. (1996). Obstetric practice and the prevalence of Urinary Incontinence three months after delivery. *Br J Obstet Gynaecol*, 103(1), 154-161.

[111] Diez-Itza, I., Ibanez, L., Arrue, M., Paredes, J., Murgiondo, A., and Sarasqueta, C. (2009). Influence of maternal weight on the new onset of stress urinary incontinence in pregnant women. *Int Urogynecol J Pelvic Floor Dysfunct*, 20, 1259–1263.

[112] Wesnes, S.L., Hunskaar, S., Bo, K., and Rortveit, G. (2010). Urinary incontinence and weight change during pregnancy and postpartum: a cohort study. *Am J Epidemiol*, 172, 1034–1044.

[113] Ruiz de Viñaspre Hernández, R., Rubio Aranda, E., and Tomás Aznar, C. (2013). Urinary incontinence and weight changes during pregnancy and post-partum: A pending challenge. *Midwifery*, 29(12), 123-9.

[114] Gunderson, E.P., Striegel-Moore, R., Schreiber, G., et al. (2009). Longitudinal study of growth and adiposity in parous compared with nulligravid adolescents. *Arch Pediatr Adolesc Med*, 163, 349–356.

[115] Walker, L.O., Fowles, E.R., and Sterling, B.S. (2011). The distribution of weight-related risks among low-income women during the first postpartum year. *J Obstet Gynecol Neonatal Nurs*, 40, 198–205.

[116] Svare, J. A., Hansen B. B. and Lose, G. (2014). Risk factors for urinary incontinence 1 year after the first vaginal delivery in a cohort of primiparous Danish women. *Int Urogynecol J*, 25, 47–51.

[117] Barbosa, A. M. P., Marini, G., Piculo, F., Rudge, C. V. C., Calderon, I. M. P., and Rudge, M. V. C. (2013). Prevalence of urinary incontinence and pelvic floor muscle dysfunction in primiparae two years after cesarean section: cross-sectional study. *Sao Paulo Med J*,131(2), 95-9.

[118] Greer, W. J., Richter, H. E., Bartolucci, A. A., and Burgio, K. L. (2008). Obesity and pelvic floor disorders: a systematic review. *Obstet Gynecol*, 112(2 Pt 1), 341-349.

[119] Bump, R. C., Sugerman, H., Fantl, J. A., and McClish, D. M. (1992). Obesity and lower urinary tract function in women: effect of surgically induced weight loss. *Am J Obstet Gynecol*, 166, 392-399.

[120] Ebbesen, M. H., Hannestad, Y. S., Midthjell, K., and Hunskaar, S. (2007). Diabetes and urinary incontinence - prevalence data from Norway. *Acta Obstet Gynecol Scand*, 86(10), 1256-1262.

[121] Dolan, L. M., Hosker, G. L., Mallett, V.T, Allen, R. E., and Smith, A. R. (2003). Stress incontinence and pelvic floor neurophysiology 15 years after the first delivery. *Br J Obstet Gynaecol*, 110, 1107-14.

[122] Gyhagen, M., Bullarbo, M., Nielsen, T., and Milsom, I. (2013). The prevalence of urinary incontinence 20 years after childbirth: a national cohort study in singleton primiparae after vaginal or caesarean delivery. *Br J Obstet Gynaecol*, 120,144-51.

[123] Liang, C. C., Chang, S. D., Lin, S. J., and Lin, Y. J. (2012). Lower urinary tract symptoms in primiparous women before and during pregnancy. *Arch Gynecol Obstet*, 285(5), 1205-1210.

[124] Arrue, M., Diez-Itza, I., Ibañez, L., Paredes, J., Murgiondo, A. and Sarasqueta, C. (2011). Factors involved in the persistence of stress urinary incontinence from pregnancy to 2 years post-partum. *Int J Gynaecol Obstet*, 115, 256–259.

[125] Subak, L.L., Wing, R., West, D.S., et al. (2009). Weight loss to treat urinary incontinence in overweight and obese women. *N Engl J Med*, 360, 481–490.

[126] Wing, R.R., West, D.S., Grady, D., et al. (2010). Effect of weight loss on urinary incontinence in overweight and obese women: results at 12 and 18 months. *J Urol*, 184, 1005–1010.

[127] Subak, L.L., Richter, H.E., and Hunskaar, S. (2009). Obesity and urinary incontinence: epidemiology and clinical research update. *J Urol*, 182, S2–S7.

[128] Hannestad, Y. S., Rortveit, G., Daltveit, A. K., and Hunskaar, S. (2003). Are smoking and other lifestyle factors associated with female urinary

incontinence? The Norwegian EPINCONT Study. *Br J Obstet Gynaecol*, 110(3), 247-254.

[129] Danforth, K. N., Townsend, M. K., Lifford, K., Curhan, G. C., Resnick, N. M., and Grodstein, F. (2006). Risk factors for urinary incontinence among middle-aged women. *Am J Obstet Gynecol*, 194(2), 339-345.

[130] Bump, R. C. and McClish, D. M. (1994). Cigarette smoking and pure genuine stress incontinence of urine: a comparison of risk factors and determinants between smokers and nonsmokers. *Am J Obstet Gynecol*, 170, 579-582.

[131] Turawa, E. B., Musekiwa, A., and Rohwer, A.C. (2014). Interventions for treating postpartum constipation. *Cochrane Database Syst Rev*, (9), CD010273.

[132] Cheng, C., and Li, Q. (2008). Integrative review of research on general health status and prevalence of common physical health conditions of women after childbirth. *Womens Health Issues*, 18(4), 267-80.

[133] Bradley, C. S., Kennedy, C. M., Turcea, A. M., Rao, S. S., and Nygaard, I. E. (2007). Constipation in pregnancy: prevalence, symptoms, and risk factors. *Obstet Gynecol*, 110(6), 1351-7.

[134] Ponce, J., Martinez, B., Fernandez, A., et al. (2008). Constipation during pregnancy: a longitudinal survey based on self-reported symptoms and the Rome II criteria. *Eur J Gastroenterol Hepatol*, 20, 56-61.

[135] van Brummen, H. J., Bruinse, H. W., van de Pol, G., Heintz, A. P., and van der Vaart, C. H. (2006). Defecatory symptoms during and after the first pregnancy: prevalences and associated factors. *Int Urogynecol J Pelvic Floor Dysfunct*, 17(3), 224-30.

[136] Shafik, A., and El-Sibai, O. (2002). Study of the levator ani muscle in the multipara: role of levator dysfunction in defecation disorders. *Obstet Gynecol*, 22(2), 187-92.

[137] Sultan, A. H., Kamm, M. A., Hudson, C. N., Thomas, J. M., and Batram, C. I. (1993). Anal-sphincter disruption during vaginal delivery. *N Engl J Med*, 329,1905-11.

[138] Penn, C., Lekan-Rutledge, D., Joers, A. M., Stolley, J. M., and Amhof, N. V. (1996). Assessment of urinary incontinence. *J Gerontol Nurs*, 22 (1), 8-19.

[139] Amselem, C., Puigdollers, A., Azpiroz, F., et al. (2010). Constipation: a potential cause of pelvic floor damage? *Neurogastroenterol Motil*, 22 (2), 150-153.

[140] Burgio, K. L., Zyczynski, H., Locher, J. L., Richter, H. E., Redden, D.T., and Wright, K. C. (2003). Urinary incontinence in the 12-month postpartum period. *Obstet Gynecol*, 102, 1291–8.

[141] Van Brummen, H. J., Bruinse, H. W., van de Pol, G., Heintz, A. P., and van der Vaart, C. H. (2007). The effect of vaginal and cesarean delivery on lower urinary tract symptoms: what makes the difference? *Int Urogynecol* J, 18,133–139.

[142] Foldspang, A., Hvidman, L., Mommsen, S., and Nielsen, J. B. (2004). Risk of postpartum urinary incon-tinence associated with pregnancy and mode of delivery. *Acta Obstet Gynecol Scand*, 83, 923–927.

[143] Viktrup, L., and Lose, G. (2001). The risk of stress incontinence 5 years after first delivery. *Am J Obstet Gynecol*, 185, 82–87.

[144] Fritel, X., Fauconnier, A., Levet, C., and Bénifla, J. L. (2004). Stress urinary incontinence 4 years after the first delivery: a retrospective cohort survey. *Acta Obstet Gynecol Scand*, 83(10), 941-945.

[145] Landon, C. R., Crofts, C. E., Smith, A. R. B., and Trowbridge, E. A. (1990). Mechanical properties of fascia during pregnancy: a possible factor in the development of stress incontinence of urine. *Contemp Rev Obstet Gynaecol*, 2, 40-46.

[146] Stainton, M. C., Strahle, A. and Fethney, J. (2005). Leaking urine prior to pregnancy: a risk factor for postnatal incontinence. *Aust N Z J Obstet Gynaecol*, 45(4), 295-299.

[147] Pizzoferrato, A. C., Fauconnier, A., Bader, G., de Tayrac, R., Fort, J., and Fritel, X. (2016). Is prenatal urethral descent a risk factor for urinary incontinence during pregnancy and the postpartum period? *Int Urogynecol J*, 27(7):1003-11.

[148] Barbosa, A. M. P., Marini, G., Piculo, F., Rudge, C. V. C., Calderon, I. M. P., and Rudge, M. V. C. (2013). Prevalence of urinary incontinence and pelvic floor muscle dysfunction in primiparae two years after cesarean section: cross-sectional study. *Sao Paulo Med J*,131(2), 95-9.

[149] Liang, C. C., Wu, M. P., Lin S. J., Lin, Y. J., Chang, S. D., and Wang, H. H. (2013). Clinical impact of and contributing factors to urinary incontinence in women 5 years after first delivery. *Int Urogynecol J*, 24, 99–104.

[150] Gartland, D., Donath, S., MacArthur, C., and Brown, S. (2012). The onset, recurrence and associated obstetric risk factors for urinary incontinence in the first 18 months after a first birth: an Australian nulliparous cohort study. *Br J Obstet Gynaecol*, 119, 1361–1369.

[151] Buchana, T. A., and Xiang, A. H. (2005). Gestational diabetes mellitus. *J Clin Invest*, 115, 485–91.

[152] Melville, J. L., Katon, W., Delaney, K., and Newton, K. (2005). Urinary incontinence in US women: a population-based study. *Arch Intern Med*, 165(5), 537-542.

[153] Saydah, S. H., Chandra, A. and Eberhardt, M. S. (2005). Pregnancy experience among women with and without gestational diabetes in the US, 1995 National survey of family growth. *Diabetes Care*, 28(5), 1035-1040.

[154] Chuang, C. M., Lin, I. F., Horng, H. C., Hsiao, Y. H., Shyu, I. L., and Chou, P. (2012). The impact of gestational diabetes mellitus on postpartum urinary incontinence: a longitudinal cohort study on singleton pregnancies. *Br J Obstet Gynecol*, 119, 1334-1343.

[155] Brown, J.S, Wessells, H., Chancellor, M. B., Howards, S., Stamm, W. E., and Stapleton, A. E. (2005). Urologic complications of diabetes. *Diabetes Care*, 28,177–85.

[156] Jackson, S. L., Scholes, D., Boyko, E. J., Abraham, L., and Fihn, S. D. (2005). Urinary incontinence and diabetes in postmenopausal women. *Diabetes Care*, 28, 1730–8.

[157] Daneshgari, F., Liu, G., Birder, G., Hanna-Mitchell, A. T., and Chacko, S. (2009). Diabetic bladder dysfunction: current translational knowledge. J Urol 182(Suppl 6), S18–26.

[158] Brown, J. S., Nyberg, L. M., Kusek, J. W., Burgio, K. L., and Diokno, A. C. (2003). Proceedings of the national institute of diabetes and digestive and kidney diseases international symposium on epidemiologic issues in urinary incontinence in women. *Am J Obstet Gynecol*, 188 (6), S77-S88.

[159] Kim, C., McEwen, L. N., Sarma, A.V., Piette, J. D., and Herman, W. H. (2008). Stress urinary incontinence in women with a history of gestational diabetes mellitus. *J. Womens Health*, 17(5), 783-792.

In: Urinary Incontinence
Editor: Debra Newton

ISBN: 978-1-53610-099-0
© 2016 Nova Science Publishers, Inc.

Chapter 3

PREDICTIVE AND BARRIER FACTORS TO TREATMENT–SEEKING BEHAVIOR AMONG WOMEN WITH URINARY INCONTINENCE

Bussara Sangsawang[1,], Nucharee Sangsawang[1] and Denchai Laiwattana[2]*

[1]Department of Maternal–Child Nursing and Midwifery Nursing, Faculty of Nursing, Srinakharinwirot University, Thailand
[2]Department of Neurosurgery, Bangkok Hospital Trat, Trat, Thailand

ABSTRACT

Urinary incontinence (UI), the complaint of involuntary loss of urine, is a common condition among women in various population ages, which has significant impact on quality of life (QoL). Estimates of the prevalence of UI vary greatly with reports ranging from approximately 2.7% to 84.12% of all women in population ages.

UI affects the QoL of women in four domains including physical activity, travel, social relationships and emotional health. Several incontinent women have responded that UI restricts lifestyles, inhibits daily activities, interferes with social activities and sexual function, and results in a loss of self-confidence. Specifically, several women who had UI symptoms have reported that UI decreases overall QoL with feelings of embarrassment, depression, anxiety, difficulty and discomfort. More

---

[*] Corresponding author: twinnui@hotmail.com.

than half (60%) of the women reported that they suffered moderate to extreme discomfort or difficulty caused by their UI symptoms.

The predicting factors of treatment-seeking behavior among incontinent women are associated with various factors such as older age, long duration and greater severity of UI symptoms with higher emotional and physical impact on QoL, more discomfort and perceived UI suffering. Women suffering from severe UI are significantly more likely to have sought treatment than those with mild to moderate UI. Therefore, the major reasons for treatment-seeking are perceived increase in severity or distress and the need for incontinence materials. In many countries, women with UI who have treatment-seeking behavior can directly visit general practitioners (GP), specialists, gynecologists or urologists to consult about their UI symptoms. However, the rate of treatment-seeking for UI is significantly lower when compared to UI prevalence. The rate of treatment-seeking behavior among incontinent women is reported at approximately 15% to 45%.

The barrier factors of treatment-seeking behavior among UI women are also associated with various factors including older age, different racial and ethnic groups, social stigmas, embarrassment about visiting healthcare providers, consideration of UI as a normal consequence of pregnancy, childbirth or aging, characteristics and types of UI, perception that UI severity is not a serious or life-threatening problem, insufficient knowledge about urinary incontinence and treatment, healthcare professionals or healthcare providers, and other factors such as perceived self-efficacy and counseling about UI symptoms from healthcare providers.

Therefore, several women tend to consider UI as a common problem in women that is inevitable with age, especially in older age. Most women who do not seek treatment do not do so because they consider their incontinence as not a very serious problem, have deficient knowledge about UI etiology and available treatments. The majority of women are not provided with information on UI by health professionals. Moreover, incontinent women who have mild symptoms of UI or do not experience daily leakage and those who do not perceive leakage as a serious troublesome with impact on their daily lives do not want treatment-seeking. The rate of non-treatment-seeking behavior among incontinent women is reported at approximately 50% to 80%. Although these women are often inconvenienced and troubled by UI symptoms, they are reluctant to seek help from health professionals. Moreover, approximately two-thirds of suffering women who do not seek help are too embarrassed to do so.

The purpose of this chapter is to review and discuss the predictive and barrier factors associated with treatment-seeking behavior among women with UI. This information can be useful for healthcare professionals when informing and counseling women who have UI to promote women's knowledge about seeking treatment for urine leakage.

INTRODUCTION

Urinary incontinence (UI), the complaint of involuntary loss of urine, is a common condition among women in various population ages across the lifespan [1]. The highest prevalence estimates found in pregnant women range from 10.8% [2] to 84.12% [3]. In postpartum women the range is from 2.7% [4] to 76.4% [5] with a range from 31.9% [6] to 62.2% [7] in adult women and from 32.2% [8] to 51.6% [9] in elderly women.

EFFECTS OF URINARY INCONTINENCE ON QUALITY OF LIFE OF WOMEN

Urinary incontinence is a common disease and significantly affects the quality of life (QoL) of women [10]. The consequences are considerable interference with social and physical activities, while the effects of UI on social life are by far greater than health-related morbidities [11]. Urinary incontinence may affect females of all ages and at all stages of life. It can also be experienced at specific times or associated with specific activities [12]. Women with UI have reported a lower QoL than women who do not experience UI [13]. Most women (30.7% to 78.0%) reported that UI had impaired QoL in terms of daily routines (praying, social activities, physical activities or sexual relationship), despite mild symptoms and with severe effects reported by 8.8% [14, 15]. Adult women are commonly affected by UI and estimations of prevalence rates vary across the literature with reports ranging anywhere from 5% to 72% [16].

Although UI does not appear to increase mortality rates, the medical morbidity substantially leads to local candida infections, cellulitis, pressure sores, constant skin irritation and sleep deprivation due to nocturia [17] associated with clinically diagnosed candidiasis (53.76%) and soreness in the perineal region (52.69%) [11].

The effects of UI on psychological morbidity include poor self-esteem, social withdrawal, depression, sexual dysfunction due to embarrassment and curtailed social and recreational activities [17]. Urinary incontinence interferes with social activities (76.34%), sexual function (22.58%) and results in despair (72.09%) [11]. In many cases, UI affects a woman's ability to take part in a variety of recreational and social activities, and has negative psychological effects including depression, anxiety and frustration [13].

For example, Lauver et al. [18] found women affected by UI to have an increased incidence of social isolation, lower stated purpose in life, less positive relations with others and increased incidence of depression. Moreover, UI has been also shown to be a barrier to social interests, physical recreation and exercise as well as other everyday activities [19]. Kumari et al. [10] found many women (70%) to report that UI affected their daily routines as well as social activities like shopping and visiting friends. Monz et al. [20] found most women to report the impact of UI symptoms on activities to affect exercise with more than 45% of women moderately to totally limited in this activity. More than half (60%) of the women reported that they were moderately to extremely bothered by their UI symptoms [20]. Saleh et al. [21] also found most of the women (62.3%) to believe that UI can cause infection, while some (20.5%) believe that it can cause skin allergy and very few think it can cause cancer or other disorders. Incontinent women who suffer are most troubled by their inability to pray (64%) and their marital relationship (47%), limitation of their social activities (20%), difficulty in doing housework (14%) and inconvenience during shopping (13%). More than half (56%) of women have found it most embarrassing to discuss UI with their husbands [21].

RATES OF TREATMENT-SEEKING BEHAVIOR AMONG WOMEN WITH URINARY INCONTINENCE

Although UI prevalence is high and UI is not considered life-threatening, the impact on an individual's QoL is tremendous, and there is an urgent need for healthcare providers to improve management of chronic conditions [11, 22]. Unfortunately, UI is a common and neglected gynecological problem with poor healthcare-seeking behavior. This health-seeking care behavior is found to be low worldwide [11] and most women with urinary incontinence (UI) do not seek professional help [23].

In many instances, Gasquet et al. [24] found only the most severely affected women who report SUI symptoms to seek help and receive treatment.

Altintas et al. [25] found a small number of patients to accept UI as a disease and search for therapy. Shaw et al. [26] found 7.7% of women to report SUI monthly or more often, and 15% of those sought help. Cooper et al. [27] found nearly half (40%) of women to suffer from UI causing significant problems at a rate of 8.5% and a total of 17% of women had sought professional help [27]. In a similar study, Hannestad et al. [28] found approximately one-quarter (26%) of incontinent women to have seen a doctor for the ailment. O'Connell et al. [29] found approximately two-thirds (31.0%) of all women to have sought help for their continence problem. Approximately 70.3% continued to have a continence problem. Of this group, 84.6% continue to be bothered by continence problem and 65.4% had taken action to treat their incontinence. Ruiz de Viñaspre Hernández et al. [30] found the treatment-seeking percentage to be 37.3% and the treatment percentage to be 27.5%. Koch [13] found less than 38% of women to have sought help for their UI symptoms. Harris et al. [31] found nearly half (45%) of women with weekly incontinence to report having ever sought care for the ailment. Of those who sought care, 60% reported receiving treatment and half of those who were treated continued to have daily leakage.

Moreover, the prevalence of older women with UI who do not seek help is high [32]. Cetinel et al. [33] found the majority of incontinent women to not seek medical help. Da Silva and Lopes [34] found a large share of the women (45.7%) to not be familiar with any form of UI treatment, while more than half (65.7%) did not seek treatment for the problem. El-Azab and Shaaban [35] found most (80%) incontinent women to have never sought medical advice.

Furthermore, incontinent women tend to delay treatment for UI. Margalith et al. [36] found the majority of the sample (74%) to delay seeking help for at least a year, while 46% delayed treatment for 3 years. Norton et al. [37] found elderly women to delay treatment for more than 5 years, while two-fifths delayed within 1 year, one-thirds delayed 1 to 5 years and one-quarter waited more than 5 years.

The many results from the abovementioned studies found only 15%–45% of all women with symptoms of incontinence to seek medical care.

Negative attitudes toward urinary incontinence treatment inhibit women in seeking care. Urinary incontinence is a stigmatized attribute [38]. This reveals that the public should be informed in detail about UI among all women in various population ages [25].

BARRIER FACTORS TO TREATMENT-SEEKING BEHAVIOR AMONG WOMEN WITH URINARY INCONTINENCE

Although there is a consensus that UI negatively affects quality of life (QOL) in women [39], the challenge to healthcare providers is that women tend to wait before seeking timely and effective treatment. Delayed treatment creates a vicious cycle for women living with UI because they attempt to adjust their lives around the ailment by restricting physical activities and enduring the psychological effects of incontinence [40].

Many studies have proposed possible reasons for the delay to treatment for UI. Existing studies have highlighted misconceptions (i.e., viewing UI as a natural outcome of aging and/or childbirth that is untreatable) [41], psychosocial barriers (shame, embarrassment, fear of discrimination) [42, 43], fear of invasive treatment and adequate self-coping strategies [44] as some of the common barriers to seeking treatment. In addition, delay to treatment for UI is common among older community-dwelling women. Margalith et al. [36] found approximately three-quarters (74.0%) of women to delay seeking help for at least 1 year, while 46% delayed for 3 years. The main reasons were insufficient time (36%), shame (15.7%) and fear of surgery in severe UI (14.7%). In Middle-Eastern women, Saleh et al. [21] indicated that UI remains underreported by Qatari women because of social and cultural attitudes and, most importantly, insufficient information, even though the ailment is relatively common in the community. In univariate and multivariate logistic regression analyses, Wu et al. [45] found the predictors of delayed treatment-seeking for UI more than 3-year to be older age (OR 1.98, 95% CI 1.31-3.00), lower subjective UI severity (OR 2.32, 95% CI 1.38-3.87) and non-mixed UI (stress [SUI] or urgency UI [UUI] only) (OR 1.60, 95% CI: 1.11-2.32).

A great deal of literature has revealed many factors to potentially act as triggers prompting women to seek help for symptoms of UI in addition to some of the barriers potentially preventing treatment-seeking behavior [12]. Understanding these reasons may help in asking specific questions during the consultation, giving those women that would like to discuss their symptoms the opportunity to do so [12].

1. Older Age

Older age is a significant predictor of longer delay to treatment in incontinent women [13, 46]. Women who are older tend to delay treatment longer. Wu et al. [45] found a longer delay to treatment-seeking behavior among older women with higher UI prevalence, which reveals the severity of under-reported UI among older women in China. The rate of healthcare-seeking behavior for UI also significantly increases with age [47]. Rios et al. [48] found younger women, association of several urinary symptoms, symptoms of urinary loss and longer time since symptom onset to be determining factors for seeking medical treatment. Minassian et al. [49] found the factors associated with health care utilization to include older age, parity (1+), number of doctor visits, urgency UI subtype, UI discomfort and impact on behavior. Similarly, Xu et al. [50] found older age and duration of urine leakage to have a negative correlation with help-seeking intentions, while educational level and previous help-seeking behaviors had a positive correlation.

2. Different Racial and Ethnic Groups

The clinical and epidemiological criteria on UI are different among diverse cultures and ethnic groups. Women across different racial and ethnic groups share similar UI management strategies and experiences. However, perceptions about UI may differ in certain populations. Across multiple studies, Siddiqui et al. [51] found women to reiterate a preference for discussing UI with other women, even if the other women were not physicians. Non-Caucasian women expressed self-blame and perceived UI as a negative outcome from childbirth or prior sexual experiences. Latina women maintained more secrecy around this issue, even amongst family members [51]. Berger et al. [52] found women across different racial and ethnic groups (African and Caucasian) to seek healthcare for UI at similarly low rates. Improved patient-doctor relationships and public education may also foster healthcare-seeking behavior [52].

With reference to QoL issues, most women affected with UI in the Middle East have different QoL concerns, including disruption of prayer schedules and interference with sexual activity [53]. Consequently, those women are expected to have different and more complex barriers than their counterparts from other cultures. The Middle Eastern culture is a male-dominated society with conservative traditions and attitudes potentially leading to unenthusiastic atmospheres toward UI [54]. Those women are underpowered minorities in their societies and are not expected to visit medical care, except in "crisis oriented" emergencies [55]. Although UI is a prevalent condition and occurs among Middle Eastern women, few women seek medical help. Only 4% of sufferers have sought medical advice compared to a relatively higher consultation rate in a European survey (31%) [56]. El-Azab, and Shaaban [35] found the barriers that prevent Middle Eastern women from seeking medical consultation for UI to be different from the barriers of women in other communities. Most common barriers include the misconceptions about the causes and availability of treatment options for UI as well as embarrassment [35].

Other factors associated with treatment-seeking include the impact of incontinence on quality of life, extent of embarrassment about talking to a physician about urinary symptoms and attitudes toward health care use [57]. Women who perceive UI as a disease and those with a higher degree of QoL impact are more likely to seek medical help. Furthermore, treatment-seeking in women with significant UI may be more common than thought as a great majority of women with higher IIQ-7 scores have been found to have sought medical help [58]. In addition, Koch [13] also found QoL scores to be another factor affecting the help-seeking behavior of women. Dunivan et al. [59] also found the greatest barriers to care-seeking for women to be related to cost and inconvenience, thereby reflecting the importance of assessing socioeconomic status when investigating barriers to care [59].

3. Social Stigma

Attitudes about seeking treatment for urinary incontinence are generally negative [38]. Several studies indicate stigma to be the main reason for not seeking treatment among UI women [35, 60]. Social stigma prevents many women from seeking treatment [22]. Stigma is defined as an attribute discrediting an individual, reducing him or her "from a hole and normal person to a tainted, discounted one" in what is typically a social process of rejection, blame or devaluation [61]. The stigmatization of physical or mental diseases involves not only the public stereotyping (i.e., social rejection, exclusion, or discrimination) of these patients but also the internalization (i.e., shame, humiliation, or embarrassment) of these stereotypes by the patients [62].

Stigma enhances the formation of negative attitudes toward seeking treatment for UI. Public stigma affects treatment-seeking attitudes through internalization of social messages [38]. For the total sample, all of the stigma domains, namely, social rejection, social isolation and internalized shame had direct negative effects on treatment-seeking attitudes [38]. The public stigma domain of social rejection also indirectly affected treatment-seeking attitudes through increasing social isolation, as well as increasing social isolation and internalized shame. The effects of internalized shame were higher in women with more severe UI [38]. In addition, stigma leading to social isolation and internalized shame negatively correlated with the QoL of patients suffering from SUI [63].

Stigma is an important factor in intentions to seek care in UI women and correlations with intentions to seek care. Wang et al. [43] found only one-third of women to intend to consult health professionals for UI during the next month. They suggested that the relationship between stigma and intentions to seek care among SUI women is complex and varies by the unique aspects of stigma. Specifically, social rejection was found to be positively correlated with intentions to seek care. In addition, women with moderate internalized shame had stronger intentions to seek care than those with low or high levels of internalized shame [43]. Moreover, the relationship of stigma with care-seeking behaviors varies with aspects of stigma and a positive pattern for social rejection with a negative quadratic pattern for internalized shame [43]. The perceived stigma mainly manifests itself as more internalized shame and less social rejection [43]. Therefore, stigma reduction strategy is aimed at promoting the use of health care targeting individuals with high internalized shame and low intentions to seek care [43].

4. Embarrassment or Shame about Visiting Healthcare Providers

Although UI is a prevalent condition and occurs among women in various population ages, few women seek medical help due to many barriers. Urinary incontinence is often stigmatized, which is a frequent reason for which patients do not seek help [64]. In addition, UI is a highly sensitive issue some women find shameful to discuss, especially those with poor educational backgrounds [35]. Therefore, embarrassment is strongly associated with reduced rates of help-seeking behavior [56, 65-67]. Moreover, embarrassment prevents some from consulting a doctor, while others believe SUI cannot be treated [68, 69]. El-Azab and Shaaban [35] found embarrassment and inadequate awareness about symptoms and availability of treatment options to be identified as barriers to help-seeking behavior [35]. Similar to what has been observed in China [63], the main reasons for not obtaining treatment are embarrassment about consulting a doctor (33.3%).

Several studies have indicated that embarrassment or shame is correlated with UI and reasons for delaying or declining to seek treatment. For example, Saleh et al. [21] found the main reason for not seeking medical attention among incontinent women to be embarrassment (40.6%) at having to speak with a doctor. Both with and without UI symptoms, the above investigators also found approximately three-quarters (70.4%) of women to believe that UI was abnormal and worth reporting to a doctor. Elbiss et al. [14] found half (50.5%) of the affected women to not seek medical advice, stating the following reasons: hope for a spontaneous resolution of UI (61.9%); embarrassment about visiting a male or female clinician (35.9%); belief that UI is a normal occurrence among women (31.5%); embarrassment about visiting a male clinician (29.3%); and no awareness that treatment was available (23.9%). Perera et al. [11] found the main reasons for not seeking medical advice to be embarrassment (33.33%) and not knowing that UI is remediable (28.40%). Roe et al. [67] also found two-thirds of sufferers to be women who did not seek help because they were too embarrassed to do so. Adedokun et al. [70] found the reasons mentioned for not seeking hospital care to include a belief that the condition is not life-threatening (51.2%), a belief that treatment is available (18.2%), insufficient funds (1.7%), shyness about disclosure (2.5%), fear of complications (1.7%) other (2.5%), and no reason (22.3%).

Margalith et al. [36] also found women who scored badly with regard to stress to be more likely to be embarrassed by their UI. Shaw et al. [71] found most women to not always communicate their concerns about urinary symptoms to their GPs due to embarrassment or misconceptions about a 'medical problem'. Hägglund and Wadensten [23] argued that the concept of incontinence being inappropriate is learnt in early childhood and is, therefore, deeply embedded.

Some factors associated with help-seeking for UI was discomfort of symptoms [40, 56, 72-75]. Discomfort is a significant because it indicates how an individual experiencing UI perceives their symptoms concerning whether they feel able to cope easily and if they find ways to cope or adopt a stoic attitude [12]. Another consistent finding reveals the severity of symptoms to not always be an indicator of how bothersome an individual perceives them to be with some women affected by a clinical definition of severe incontinence, not reporting discomfort and, conversely, some with mild symptoms reporting that their symptoms bothered them sufficiently that they sought help [40, 56, 72-75]. Cetinel et al. [33] found only 12% of incontinent women to have previously sought medical help for their problem. They also found frequency, severity and type of UI to be independent factors for predicting bothersome UI, while only discomfort increased help-seeking behavior.

5. Considering Urinary Incontinence as a Normal Consequence of Pregnancy, Childbirth or Aging

Generally, most women tend to consider UI as a normal part of childbirth or aging [71]. A toning down and minimization of UI problems is associated with incontinence as the ailment is considered a normal consequence of pregnancy and childbirth [23]. Mason et al., [40] found women to feel that SUI could occur during pregnancy or following childbirth and women generally felt embarrassed to talk about the condition, while some women felt their problem was minimal or that they could cope with it. Therefore, these findings suggest the roles of various healthcare professionals and whether or not midwives or health visitors might be well-placed in advising pregnant and postpartum women regarding UI. Furthermore, healthcare professionals should ask about symptoms rather than the women having to mention the presence of these themselves [12].

Similarly, the misconception that UI is a normal part of aging causes older women to frequently regard incontinence as a normal consequence of aging [76]. Women perceive UI as a part of the natural aging process in which low successful treatment and low rates of treatment-seeking behavior [27]. Therefore, the commonly held belief that the occurrence of UI is a normal part of aging can act as a barrier to seeing help [65, 66, 73]. Individuals tend to normalize their symptoms and accept deterioration as an inevitable part of getting older [12]. Dispelling this misconception and raising awareness that developing urinary symptoms is not an inevitable part of aging, but an ailment for which treatments can be highly effective would appear to be an important message [12].

The belief that UI symptoms may improve with time [37] and are not regarded as abnormal or serious problems [68, 77, 78] are the main reasons women do not seek treatment. In a community-based descriptive cross-sectional study, Hemachandra et al. [79] found the barriers to healthcare to include fear of vaginal examination, shame and embarrassment with a belief that SUI is a natural consequence of aging and childbirth. Kumari et al. [10] also found the most common reason quoted for not seeking treatment to be, 'UI is considered 'normal', 'did not take it seriously' and 'shyness.' Perera et al. [11] found that perceiving SUI to be a normal consequence of childbirth was the main reason for not seeking medical advice. Similarly, El-Azab and Shaaban [35] found a common barrier to seeking help for UI symptoms to be assuming UI as a normal part of aging and embarrassment.

Of the incontinent women in the sample group, Ng et al. [15] found more than half (52.9%) to think incontinence was inevitable with age, 22.2% to believe that they should cope with the problem themselves, 13.7% to think that no useful treatment was available and only 3.9% to have sought medical advice before. Kinchen et al. [57] found women seeking health care to also be less likely to be embarrassed about talking to health professionals and less likely to accept urinary incontinence as 'normal'. After delivery, the women did not expect the UI problems to be so severe. They hoped their problems would improve spontaneously. The women talked to close relatives and acquaintances (female relatives and friends who had had deliveries themselves), who confirmed that the problems were an inevitable consequence of vaginal delivery and that there were no real treatment options [80].

Higa and Lopes [81] found the most common reasons for not seeking treatment to be that incontinence was mild (28.8%) and the belief that the UI was a common problem for women (22%). The prevalence and reasons for not seeking treatment for UI were similar to other researches on women in general. It was concluded that the factor of health professionals did not influence attitudes [81].

6. Characteristics and Types of Urinary Incontinence

Urinary incontinence characteristics were most strongly associated with treatment-seeking behavior in midlife women [82]. In multivariable analyses, Waetjen et al. [82] found women to have higher odds of seeking treatment when UI symptoms were more frequent (adjusted OR 3.16, 95% CI 1.15-8.67) and more bothersome (adjusted OR 1.09, 95% CI 1.01-1.18), with longer symptom duration and worsening UI symptoms (adjusted OR 1.75, 95% CI

1.01-3.04) in the year before treatment was sought. In addition, types of UI such as SUI, UUI and MUI were also associated with seeking health behavior. Wu et al. [45] found women who reported SUI or UUI alone to have longer delays in seeking treatment compared to women with mixed UI [45]. This could be explained in that women with mixed UI symptoms typically describe more severe and troublesome incontinence than women with only one type of UI [83]. Therefore, this implies that community health professionals should prioritize interventions for incontinent women based on UI type. Furthermore, women who report SUI or UUI should be targeted for education and intervention [45].

7. Perceived Urinary Incontinence Severity is not a Serious or Life-Threatening Problem

The major reasons for seeking help were perceived increase in UI severity or distress and the need for incontinence materials [84]. Therefore, perceived UI severity is a predictor of help-seeking behavior in incontinent women [13]. Wu et al. [45] found lower subjective UI severity or lower perceived UI severity to contribute to longer delay to UI treatment. Hagglund et al. [85] also found women who sought professional help to have more severe urine leakage than those who did not seek help. Similarly, Teunissen et al. [84] found most patients who had not sought help did not do so because they considered incontinence as not being very serious, or due to deficient knowledge about cause and treatment options - comments such as 'incontinence is age-related', and 'there is nothing that can be done about incontinence', were reported.

In postnatal women, Perera et al. [11] found the main reasons for not seeking medical advice to include perceiving SUI to be a normal consequence of childbirth (23.46%) and having to attend to needs of the family (14.81%). In addition, none who had been pregnant (n = 313) had received advice on postnatal pelvic floor exercises [11].

El-Azab and Shaaban [35] found women to perceive UI as an aging phenomenon rather than a pathological condition caused by childbirth or menopause. Therefore, symptoms are sometimes not felt to be very serious, while help-seeking should be reserved for more serious conditions. Interestingly, the investigators found the factors strongly promoting women to seek consultation to be spousal encouragement, followed by prayer affection for Muslims, and incontinence severity [35]. The factors that promoted women in the US were different, including symptom duration >3 years, having a history of noticeable accidents, worse QoL scores, not being embarrassed to talk with a physician about urinary symptoms, talking with others about UI, and keeping regular appointments for routine/preventive care [57].

This is consistent with available data from Northern Europe [86]. With regard to the severity of UI, only 26.9% of women had mild UI and the majority (73.1%) had moderate to severe incontinence when assessed using the UI severity scale. High percentage of moderate to severe UI together with very poor treatment-seeking behavior may be responsible for the complications experienced by the study group [86].

Considering these factors, it is understandable that women who report being less severely troubled by UI symptoms report longer delay to treatment and that they believe they can manage UI successfully without additional assistance [85].

8. Insufficient Knowledge about Urinary Incontinence and Treatment

Insufficient knowledge of the etiology and treatment of UI can be a barrier to help-seeking and successful outcome [87]. Da Silva and Lopes [34] found insufficient knowledge about the types of treatment can contribute to not seeking professional help. Therefore, raising awareness among patients may represent the greatest opportunity to help patients with symptoms of UI [12].

9. Healthcare Professionals or Healthcare Providers

The majority of women are not provided with information on UI symptoms but they want health professionals to provide a warning that UI conditions could occur. They also wanted health professionals to seek out information about symptoms rather than the women themselves having to broach the subject [40]. Shaw et al. [71] found the most common theme to emerge to be insufficient knowledge of the UI condition and inadequately available treatments.

Most women are reluctant to seek help for treatment of UI, even though they are often inconvenienced and troubled by the condition [40, 88]. Kinchen et al. [57] found only 38% of women with UI symptoms to have initiated conversation with physicians about incontinence. There are two main reasons for women's reluctance to seek help [40]. First, the women feel they do not need help (or do not want to admit they need help). Some women report that the condition causes no problems [40], believing SUI to be a normal consequence of childbirth [89]. Therefore they had no reason to seek help. Second, the women did not want to discuss the condition with a health care professional [40]. The women regarded the condition as something of a taboo and were embarrassed by having it or even talking about it in many cases. Therefore, some women are reluctant to discuss their condition with some health professionals, but would welcome the opportunity to discuss their problem with someone [40].

The reluctance to seek professional help appears to be exacerbated by the nature of the women's relationships with some health professionals and a minority of women feels that certain health professionals, usually their GPs, are unapproachable [40]. Other women worry about their reactions, assuming that their condition will be perceived as a minor problem and a waste of their GP's time [40]. Therefore, the GP does not seem to be the choice of the women for discussing such topics as stress incontinence [40].

Unfortunately, studies exploring physicians' responses to consultation for incontinence also show their responses to be unsatisfactory, even with older women and other types of incontinence [40]. These findings may suggest that health professionals need to initiate the conversation. When health professionals make general inquiries after a woman's health, it is seen as a polite gesture to approach conversation about UI [40].

Women's reluctance is reluctant to discuss UI symptoms with health care providers could be improved by careful handling and a good relationship with the patient. In this way, issues of embarrassment could be minimized [12]. When women are not reluctant to seek help, they will seek treatment for their UI symptoms from health professionals. Waetjen et al. [82] found women who saw physicians regularly and received more preventive women's health advice at visits, or both, were more likely to seek UI treatment (adjusted OR 1.18, 95% CI 1.07, 1.30).

10. Other Factors

In addition, other factors such as perceived self-efficacy and counseling about UI symptoms from healthcare providers can contribute the predictors for seeking treatment behavior. Perceived self-efficacy is a negative predictor, while perceived social impact is a positive predictor. Wu et al. [42] found the resultant model to demonstrate that incontinent women's help-seeking intention could be predicted by their perceived self-efficacy and perceived social impact from urine loss. Overall, the predictive model explained 36% of the variance for incontinent women's help-seeking intentions [42].

In multiple logistic regressions, the findings of Ruiz de Viñaspre Hernández et al. [30] indicated that counseling about UI in pregnancy, postpartum physical exercise and Spanish nationality predicted 47.8% of the variance in treatment-seeking behavior. Moreover, they also found the absence of counseling to largely determine low rates of treatment-seeking among Spanish mothers [30].

SELF-CARE STRATEGIES TO MANAGE URINARY INCONTINENCE SYMPTOMS

Normalizing UI can be seen as just one way of coping and protecting oneself [23]. Individuals who do not seek help for their urinary symptoms are more likely to adopt coping and avoidance strategies [90]. Porrett and Cox [64] suggest that women with UI create their own set of behaviors to cope. Some women may feel less troubled by UI than others because they believe that they can successfully manage their symptoms independently [91]. Therefore, both young and old women tend to conceal UI in their daily lives by keeping the bladder empty, limiting social interactions and using hygienic measures [92].

Berger et al. [52] found women across different racial and ethnic groups (African and Caucasian) to be similar in percentage, use of medications and some self-care strategies such as pad wearing and bathroom mapping, but women of African ethnicity were significantly more likely to restrict fluid intake than Caucasian women and marginally less likely to perform Kegels.

Saleh et al. [21] found coping mechanisms among incontinent women in the Middle East to include frequent washing (58.3%), wearing a protective perennial pad (42.4%), changing underwear frequently (41.3%), decreasing fluid intake (19.8%) and stopping all work (4.9%). Moreover, Papanicolaou et al. [93] found most of the women to use protective pads, whereby more than half of the patients paid out-of-pocket, despite potential healthcare reimbursement schemes.

PREDICTIVE FACTORS TO TREATMENT-SEEKING BEHAVIOR AMONG WOMEN WITH URINARY INCONTINENCE

The predicting factors of treatment-seeking behavior among incontinent women are associated with various factors such as older age, long duration and greater severity of UI symptoms, greater emotional and physical impact on QoL with more discomfort and perceived UI suffering.

1. Older Age

Apart from UI severity and type, care-seeking behavior is associated with aging [94]. The care-seeking behavior rate increases with age [94]. Older age and high impact of symptoms are the factors most strongly associated with help-seeking [28]. Margalith et al. [36] found older age, psychological stress, perceived suffering and social functioning to be associated with care-seeking patterns. Similarly, Visser et al. [32] found care-seeking behavior to be associated with increasing age and higher levels of distress caused by the symptoms. Younger patients more frequently hesitate to consult their GPs if they perceive their symptoms to be relatively mild [32].

2. Duration, Severity and Types of Urinary Incontinence

Women with high incontinence impact and symptom distress are more likely to seek treatment than those with lower impact and symptom distress [95]. Hannestad et al. [28] found increasing age, impact, severity and duration to all be significantly associated with consultation rates, as urge and mixed types are compared with stress incontinence, as well as having visited any doctor during the previous 12 months. Fifty percent of the women with significant incontinence (moderate/severe incontinence perceived as troublesome) had seen a doctor because of their incontinence [28].

Moreover, the category or type of UI may affect the likelihood of seeking help [26, 56, 75, 96]. Women with mixed urinary incontinence (MUI) and urged urinary incontinence (UUI) to be those most likely to consult with a health care provider about their symptoms [26, 75, 96]. However, the reason for this was not explored and might be explained by other factors such as UUI becoming more prevalent with increased age and help-seeking behavior also being more likely in older age groups [12].

3. Perceived Severity of Urinary Incontinence

A statistically significant association was found between the severity of UI symptoms and help-seeking behavior for treatment [97]. Help-seeking behavior is influenced by the severity of incontinence [67]. Women who suffer from severe UI and have greater impact on QoL are more likely to have sought treatment than those women with mild to moderate UI [26]. Andersson et al. [97] found the perceived severity of UI to determine whether afflicted persons seek treatment or not. Persons who do not experience daily leakage and those who do not perceive the leakage as troublesome or having an effect on their daily lives mostly stated that they did not seek treatment [97].

Fritel et al. [94] found multivariate analysis to show that women who reported severe UI (OR = 4.1; 95% CI 2.6-6.5), mixed UI (2.0; 1.3-3.0), or neurologic disease (1.6; 1.1-2.6), had weak social support (1.4; 1.0-2.0), or talked about their UI with close friends or family members (1.5; 1.0-2.1) to be more likely to seek care for UI. Roe et al. [67] found the majority of sufferers to have mentioned or contacted their GP about their incontinence, and that people currently suffering from incontinence are significantly more likely to have seen their GP within the last month than those who are continent. Teunissen et al. [84] found help-seeking to be related to the duration of symptoms, the severity of incontinence, the emotional and and/or physical impact with the presence of concomitant symptoms, particularly of urinary obstruction.

4. Having Spoken to Family and Close Friends about Urinary Incontinence Symptoms

According to O'Donnell et al. [56] UI and women's attitudes were found to be associated with help-seeking after adjusting women's age, UI duration and frequency and 'discomfort' of UI; factors traditionally associated with help-seeking. After adjusting for these factors, willingness to take long-term medication and having spoken to others about UI were found to be strong predictors of help-seeking.

Apart from UI severity and type, care-seeking behavior is also associated with aging, weak social support, conversation about with close friends and family members and neurologic disorders [94]. El-Azab and Shaaban [35] found the factors significantly associated with seeking help to be spousal encouragement, prayer affection and severe UI. Furthermore, help-seeking behavior often depends on beliefs about UI and an understanding of how the condition can be treated [98].

5. Extent of Embarrassment about Talking with Healthcare Providers Concerning Urinary Incontinence Symptoms

Other factors associated with treatment-seeking also include the impact of incontinence on QoL, extent of embarrassment about talking to a physician about urinary symptoms and attitudes toward healthcare use [57]. Therefore, the findings of the study of Bradway and Strumpf [99] suggest that women who seek care for UI are more likely than those who do not seek care to 1) tell a story; 2) describe UI as having a negative impact on sense of self and 3) be older, Caucasian, in "good" or "excellent" general health, and have suffered from UI for a longer period of time than those who choose not to seek care. In a multivariate logistic regression analysis, Kinchen et al. [57] found some of the factors significantly correlated with treatment-seeking to be symptom duration >3 years (OR 2.33, 95% CI 1.57-3.45), a history of noticeable accidents (OR 1.41, 95% CI 1.06-1.87), worse disease-specific QoL scores (OR 1.89, 95% CI 1.32-2.70), no embarrassment about talking with a physician about urinary symptoms (OR 1.65, 95% CI 1.28-2.14), talking with others about UI (OR 3.34, 95% CI 2.49-4.49) and keeping regular appointments for routine/preventive care (OR 2.25, 95% CI 1.54-3.29).

In many countries, women with UI who have treatment-seeking behavior can directly visit general practitioners (GP), specialists, gynecologists, urologists, nurses, midwives and health care providers to consult about their UI symptoms.

Kumari et al. [10] found one-fifth (20%) of women to have consulted some health agency. However, only (8.6%) of women had heard about pelvic floor muscle exercises (PFME). Teunissen et al. [84] found half of the women to have sought help from a GP. Shaw et al. [26] found most (78%) women to have spoken to their GP, and 77% to have received some form of treatment or advice, but only 35% to have received recommended treatments. Papanicolaou et al. [93] found women in Spain and Germany to be more likely to have consulted a specialist for their UI symptoms; this had implications for utilization of diagnostic procedures. Conservative treatment, particularly pelvic floor muscle exercises, was more common in patients in the UK/Ireland treated in primary care by GPs.

Among women with UI, one half has discussed their incontinence with a health care provider and one third has received some form of treatment. Melville et al. [100] found half (50%) of women to have discussed their incontinence with a health care provider, 21% to have reported receiving surgery or prescription medication, 10% to have reported performing PFME and 48% to have reported wearing a pad to absorb urine daily or weekly. The following factors were significantly associated with the odds for discussing UI with a health care provider such as the following: 1) age [50 to 69 years, adjusted odds ratio 1.5 [1.1 to 2.0]; 70 to 89 years, adjusted odds ratio 1.9 [1.4, 2.7]), 2) duration of UI (2 to 5 years, adjusted odds ratio 1.9 [1.3 to 2.8]; more than 5 years, adjusted odds ratio 2.8 [2.0, 4.1]), 3) severe UI (adjusted odds ratio 1.7 [1.2 to 2.6]); and 4) greater effect on daily activities (adjusted odds ratio 2.7 [1.9, 3.8]) [100].

In addition, older women were found to be more likely to adapt to their symptoms and learn to live with them rather than "bother" their general practitioner with their problem. Kinchen et al. [57] found less than half of the women who reported symptoms of UI to have talked with their health care providers about their symptoms.

Kinchen et al. [57] found approximately one-third (38%) of women to have initiated a conversation with a physician about incontinence. Less than half of community-dwelling adult U.S. women with symptoms of UI have talked with a physician about urinary incontinence. Yip et al. [101] found women who sought medical advice from general practitioners in which 38.2% sought advice from private specialists, 17.6% from public hospitals and 2.9% from Chinese herbalists. In contrast, most women who not sought medical advice (94.4%) did not think their symptoms were serious, 8.7% did not know help was available and 3.2% claimed they had no time.

In pregnant and postpartum women, Sangi-Haghpeykar et al. [102] found most women to not readily disclose information regarding incontinence to their medical providers. Therefore, health professionals such as midwives or health visitors should be identified as the main care providers during the antenatal and postnatal periods [40]. For the participants' preference of personal sources for help with UI, the discussion about UI is a private issue for women who feel most comfortable discussing SUI with nurses and midwives [103] and find midwives to be the health care professionals who most commonly provide women with information about UI (33%) and PFME (55%) during the antenatal and postnatal periods.

In addition, women generally perceive the information as being helpful in which the information from physiotherapists obtained the highest mean ratings for helpfulness [103]. It would seem that nurses and midwives need to take responsibility for giving women this information as a matter of routine postpartum care [104].

Participants indicate group classes to be their least preferred form of help. Therefore, it may be best for health care professionals to raise the topic of UI in private consultations with pregnant and postpartum women [103]. Whitford et al. [105] found few women (21.8%) to report having received information about pelvic floor exercises during pregnancy from a midwife, possibly because midwives regard the encouragement to perform pelvic floor exercises as a recommendation from a physiotherapist. Only 8.4% of women report receiving information from a physiotherapist (not including women who gained information from a physiotherapist during a parent education class).

Generally, women have no contact with a physiotherapist during pregnancy (except when they attend parent education classes or have a physical problem necessitating referral). Consequently, women do not receive this information [105].

In addition, women in the postpartum period indicate that they would also prefer to consult with continence nurses or general nurses if they experience UI. Therefore, health care professionals do not consistently provide postpartum women with information on UI and PFME [103].

This means discussing issues in such a way that pregnant and postpartum women feel comfortable about discussing adherence problems with the midwives [104]. Therefore, it is pleasing that most research demonstrates that pregnant women view midwives as health professionals to whom they are most likely to be able to disclose information or seek consultations about UI [104].

In contrast, Rozensky et al. [106] found 13.01% of women to not have spoken to a healthcare provider about their UI symptoms, while 24.73% had never seen a healthcare professional who "specializes in bladder problems," and 75% said they were not currently using any active approach to manage symptoms, providing the reason that use of such information is discussed in terms of how to construct internet healthcare information to maximize seeking appropriate healthcare services and preparing internet-based information regarding incontinence diagnosis and treatment.

However, the rate of treatment-seeking for UI was significantly lower when compared to the prevalence of UI. The rate of treatment-seeking behavior among incontinent women is reported by approximately 15% to 45%.

STRATEGIES FOR PROMOTING WOMEN'S TREATMENT-SEEKING BEHAVIOR FOR URINARY INCONTINENCE

Help-seeking behavior often depends on beliefs about UI and an understanding of how the condition can be treated [98]. Therefore, beliefs about UI and understanding the ways in which the condition can be treated are important factors in seeking help [98].

Health education, increasing awareness to seek health care, increasing awareness with regard to UI and the training of health professionals are required to improve the understanding of women's experiences about UI symptoms and develop appropriate services with which to manage this condition [98].

Health education is paramount to women's awareness of what help is available. On an individual level, nurses have a role to play in encouraging women to seek help and making them aware of the condition as well as treatment options available to manage symptoms [98].

As previously mentioned above, most research has been found to demonstrate that women receive information about UI from a number of medical professionals such as midwives, nurses, physicians, GPs, or physiotherapists, thereby showing that the duty of providing this information to incontinent women is not exclusive to any particular person.

Regardless, the duty should belong to all medical personnel providing care for women in various population ages such as pregnant women, postpartum women, adult women and elderly women, which also include nurses or midwives.

Therefore, nurses or midwives who are considered to be the medical personnel most closely working with all women should apply this information to the care of all women and part of this role should also be adjusted to nursing practice as follows:

1. Nursing Roles

Facilitating proper treatment is a key role for health professionals. Da Silva and Lopes [34] and Shaw et al. [72] indicate that some women failed to receive treatment when presenting symptoms to their health professionals because they were told to return when the symptoms had worsened. Therefore, nurses have an important role to play in challenging the myths and breaking down the barriers that prevent women from seeking help for this condition [98].

2. Increasing Awareness to Seek Health Care

Seeking help is particularly determined by the impact experienced and presence of concomitant symptoms. When patients perceive their incontinence as not very serious or distressing and have deficient knowledge about cause and treatment options, they usually refrain from seeking help. When they perceive an increase in severity or distress, or require incontinence materials, they usually do seek help [84]. Concerns about the meaning of incontinence for overall and future health are important reasons for women choosing to seek treatment [57].

Alewijnse et al. [107] found the majority of women with UI to fail to seek help due to feelings of shame, deficient knowledge about management options or viewpoints that UI is an inevitable condition after delivery with symptoms increasing with age. Thus, it is important that health professionals ask about symptoms of SUI if women have potential risk factors for developing SUI.

Embarrassment was strongly associated with reduced rates of help-seeking behavior [56, 65-67]. Embarrassment about discussing UI symptoms with health care providers can be improved by a careful handling and good relationship with the patient [12].

Disseminating knowledge to communities to help remove the stigma of UI is an important component of this effort. Patient-centered interventions involve explaining, counseling and building skills to help patients adopt health-related behaviors and encourage change [18]. Robinson et al. [12] have found women to be more likely to seek help if they attended more visits to a health-care provider or spoke to others. By raising awareness about UI, healthcare professionals can help women realize that they are not alone in experiencing urinary symptoms. This may help in removing some of the stigma and may encourage women to ask for help and advice [12].

Social stigma prevents many women from seeking treatment, and healthcare providers often have inadequate time to inquire about bladder health [22]. Therefore, stigma reduction may help incontinent women form positive treatment-seeking attitudes and engage them in treatment [38]. Therefore, interventions should specifically target the self-stigma domains of social isolation and internalized shame in women with UI to most efficiently increase their use of health care [38].

High perceived self-efficacy in dealing with incontinent symptoms could hinder incontinent women from seeking help from healthcare providers. The strong social impact women perceive, however, facilitates intention to seek help. Therefore, nurses should understand and address these factors through education and evidence-based practices to increase help-seeking in incontinent women.

In pregnant women, midwives or nurses need to first admit that UI frequently encountered during pregnancy is not a normal condition. Rather, UI is an abnormal condition. If encountered in any woman during pregnancy with no risks for weakening the pelvic floor muscles, PFME will help minimize risks and be able to prevent UI during pregnancy [104].

In older women, healthcare providers should be aware that some women hold such beliefs and provide information about evidence-based self-management strategies or encourage older women to seek professional treatment [45]. In addition, based on the chronic progressive process of UI, older women with lower subjective UI severity and SUI or UUI alone should be targeted for community health education and intervention to promote timely treatment for UI [45].

Moreover, the theory of planned behavior can be used to predict help-seeking intention in women with UI [42]. Community nurses should increase patients' help-seeking intention by addressing perceived social impact and perceived self-efficacy in managing incontinent symptoms [42].

3. Increasing Awareness about Urinary Incontinence

Insufficient awareness of UI can be improved by simply asking about urinary symptoms in the same way as other conditions and with follow-up advice and sign-posting about other sources of information or local services [12]. Health education about UI from various health professionals has a key role to play in breaking down misconceptions about UI and increasing women's knowledge of treatment options [98]. This health education may improve women's awareness in an environment where help-seeking from health professionals is available.

There are needs for improved and widespread education to help women better understands the physiological changes involved in the development of UI [108]. Through continence education, women can be encouraged to engage in preventive activities, or take charge of the problem and work toward management or cure [108]. A proactive approach to continence education that involves individual patients as well as the community is critical to decreasing the barriers associated with access to health care services and increasing early intervention for UI [108].

In fact, the type of UI is a positive predictor for help-seeking and could be linked to other factors such as increased discomfort, greater likelihood for co-morbidities or greater impact on QoL. The above factor is worth considering when asking about symptoms and the potential impact of the aforementioned on the women affected [12].

On an individual level, nurses have a role to play in encouraging women to seek help, and making them aware of the condition and treatment options available to manage symptoms [98]. Bradway et al. [22] suggested that nurses play a role in driving this response by increasing awareness of LUTS such as UI, taking the lead in examining barriers to treatment, and providing long-term support for patients.

For pregnant and postpartum women, the women are not motivated to seek professional help. However, the women do indicate that they require professional information about their pelvic floor problems but were ashamed to talk about them [80]. Midwives should correct misunderstandings about UI in pregnant women who understand that UI is a normal occurrence during pregnancy that will disappear postpartum without seeking treatment, or that UI is either unavoidable or untreatable [104]. Therefore, if midwives discover any pregnant women to have symptoms of UI, the midwives should advise the pregnant women that having UI is neither embarrassing nor disgusting [104]. Hence, pregnant women should not be embarrassed about receiving consultation from health care professionals or avoid treatment for the symptoms occurring [104].

Pregnant women should choose to consult health care professionals they trust or with whom they feel comfortable about sharing this information. Midwives are ready to provide this information to all pregnant women [104]. In addition, midwives or nurses should possess knowledge about UI and UI prevention by various methods, particularly treatment by PFME which is accepted as the best method for preventing and treating UI during pregnancy in order to enable the provision of accurate information for pregnant women in the future [104]. Consequently, nursing information about pelvic floor problems after childbirth from midwives during pregnancy can substantially contribute to increasing the number of women treated for postpartum UI [30]. Therefore, health professionals caring for women during pregnancy or following childbirth need to raise awareness of the condition, available treatment and pro-activity in seeking out women experiencing incontinence rather than expecting women to approach them for help [40].

Unfortunately, postpartum women are uninformed about pelvic floor problems after childbirth. Therefore, the women need to discuss their pelvic floor dysfunction with close relatives and acquaintances who feed their hope that the problems will resolve spontaneously [80]. Buurman and Lagro-Janssen [80] found that postpartum women want to understand their problems and know how to deal with them. Therefore, the postpartum period is a time for obstetricians and midwives to focus on the mother's health after delivery so mothers will suffer less from pelvic floor problems, have greater awareness of what they can do about them and call in medical aid [80].

On a community level, community based education may help minimize the occurrence, and improve the quality of life of those affected [11]. The public should be educated to seek care for urine leakage, health care providers should take the initiative to ask their patients about urinary symptoms and give more attention to ensuring that treatment provided is appropriate and effective [31].

Therefore, providing adequate knowledge for women about UI through health education would improve knowledge on prevention and available treatment options. This may change the perceptions of women on UI leading to better QoL of the affected population [11]. It is also recommended that assessment of urinary incontinence include a description of the effects of UI on the physical, psychological and social domains of health, even at the primary level evaluation when UI is suspected [11].

4. Training for Health Professionals

Women need the opportunity to discuss symptoms and ensure that appropriate treatment is provided [98]. The NICE guidelines [109] set out a clear framework for assessing the physical symptoms of UI. However, there is a clear need for additional education among health professionals concerning the holistic treatment of women with UI and the importance of contextual and psychological factors [109].

In middle-aged and elderly women, UI is a condition afflicting many individuals seeking outpatient physical therapy beyond those seeking care for UI. Using simple screening to measure for UI and its impact on HR QoL is recommended as part of a routine initial evaluation in outpatient physical therapy settings [110].

During pregnancy and the postpartum period, primary prevention of UI should be encouraged with increased public awareness about pelvic floor exercises to increase the pelvic floor muscle strength, particularly during and after pregnancy. The aforementioned practice would definitely help reduce the prevalence of UI [11]. This aspect should be further emphasized in the curricula of relevant health professionals such as midwives. In Sri Lanka primary health care workers (who are mostly women) work closely with the community concerning healthcare services and health education at the grass root level [11]. It is important to assess the knowledge, beliefs and attitudes of these healthcare staff regarding UI as doing so will influence patients' perceptions of UI. In this regard, further research is recommended to assess the knowledge and attitudes of primary care health staff as the findings of such studies would have a direct impact on the care provided for women [11].

Therefore, nurses or midwives should adjust the methods employed in providing information about UI and PFME as suitable for the characteristics of regular daily work, possibly beginning by screening for UI risk factors for all pregnant women receiving antenatal services in order to assess which pregnant women are at risk for developing SUI during pregnancy. In addition, midwives should provide additional instructions about UI and PFME as another topic apart from the instructions for self-care during pregnancy. In doing so, every pregnant woman should be instructed about issues such as food intake, adequate rest, exercise and keeping antenatal appointments [104].

In this way, the guidelines for providing instructions about UI and PFME could be easily provided without disturbing the regular workloads of midwives because implementation would only involve adding this content to the content midwives already regularly provide for pregnant women [104].

Sangi-Haghpeykar et al. [102] suggested that the routines and universal counseling concerning risks for SUI and the efficacy of PFME should become an integral part of antenatal or postpartum care before hospital discharge with emphasis on the importance of designing an exercise program that can be easily incorporated into the daily routines of new mothers [111].

The instructions could be provided routinely as part of antenatal care rather than during antenatal or other voluntary classes attended only by a proportion of the women [104]. The responsibility for the task may be best held by the midwives as they provide care for women during pregnancy when the women suggest that information should be given. However, it might be useful to adopt a multidisciplinary approach with respect to reminding women to perform pelvic floor exercises [104].

CONCLUSION

Urinary incontinence is a common condition among women in various population ages across the lifespan. The highest prevalence estimates found in pregnant women range from 10.8% [2] to 84.12% [3], with a range of 2.7% [4] to 76.4% [5] in postpartum women, 31.9% [6] to 62.2% [7] in adult women and 32.2% [8] to 51.6% [9] in elderly women. Therefore, estimates of the prevalence of UI vary greatly with reports ranging from approximately 2.7% to 84.12% of all women in population ages.

It is well-known that UI is related to the weakening of the pelvic floor muscle strength, connective tissues and fascia as well as their supportive and sphincteric function. When the urethral pressure becomes less than bladder pressure and intra-abdominal pressure, the result is urethral sphincter incompetence. If the urethral sphincter is not strong enough to close the urethra, the consequence is urine leakage.

Urinary incontinence is a common disease and significantly affects the QoL of women. Women with UI have reported a lower QoL than women who do not experience UI. Urinary incontinence also interferes with social activities, sexual function and results in despair. In many cases, UI affects a woman's ability to take part in a variety of recreational and social activities, and has negative psychological effects including depression, anxiety and frustration.

Unfortunately, UI is a common and neglected gynecological problem with poor healthcare-seeking behavior. The health seeking care behavior is found to be low worldwide. Most women with urinary incontinence (UI) do not seek professional help. The researchers found only 15%–45% of all women with symptoms of incontinence to seek medical care.

Delay or not treatment-seeking behavior creates a vicious cycle for women living with UI. Many studies have proposed possible reasons for the delay to treatment for UI. Understanding these reasons may help ask specific questions during the consultation, giving those women who would like to discuss their symptoms the opportunity to do so. Based on the findings, barrier factors to treatment-seeking behavior among UI women are also associated with various reasons including older age, different racial and ethnic groups, social stigma, embarrassment about visiting healthcare providers, considering UI as a normal consequence of pregnancy and childbirth or aging, characteristics and types of UI, perceived severity that UI is not a serious or life-threatening problem, insufficient knowledge about UI and treatment, healthcare professional or healthcare providers and other factors such as perceived self-efficacy and counseling about UI symptoms from healthcare provider.

Individuals who do not seek help for their urinary symptoms are more likely to adopt coping and avoidance strategies. Some women may feel less troubled by UI than others because they believe they can successfully manage their symptoms independently. Therefore, both young and old women tend to conceal urinary incontinence in their daily lives by keeping the bladder empty, limiting social interactions, using hygiene measures, wearing a protective perennial pad, changing underwear frequently and restricting fluid intake with marginally less likelihood of performing pelvic floor muscle exercises.

The predicting factors of treatment-seeking behavior among incontinent women are associated with various factors. Based on the findings, the predicting factors of treatment-seeking behavior among UI women are older age, long duration and greater severity of UI symptoms, perceived UI suffering, having spoken to family and close friends about urinary incontinence symptoms and extent of embarrassment about talking with healthcare providers about UI symptoms. Women suffering from significantly severe UI are more likely to have sought treatment than those with mild to moderate UI. In many countries, women with UI who have treatment-seeking behavior can directly visit general practitioners (GP), specialists, gynecologists or urologists to consult about their UI symptoms. However, the rate of treatment-seeking for UI is significantly lower when compared to the prevalence of UI. The rate of treatment-seeking behavior among incontinent women is reported by approximately 15% to 45%.

Help-seeking behavior often depends on beliefs about UI and an understanding of how the condition can be treated. Health education, increasing awareness about seeking health care, increasing awareness about UI and training health professionals are required to improve the understanding of women's experiences about UI symptoms and develop appropriate services with which to manage this condition. Nurses or midwives, who are considered to be the medical personnel most closely working with all women, should apply this information to the care of all women and part of this role should also be applied to nursing practice as follows: 1) nursing roles, 2) increasing awareness about seeking health care, 3) increasing awareness about urinary incontinence and 4) training health professionals.

In addition, these health care professionals need to be regularly updated with new information and encouraged to communicate with others in the ongoing care of women over the lifespan.

REFERENCES

[1]   Haylen, B. T., de Ridder, D., Freeman, R. M., et al. (2010). An International Urogynecological Association (IUGA)/International Continence Society (ICS) joint report on the terminology for female pelvic floor dysfunction. *Int Urogynecol J*, *21*(1), 5–26.

[2]   Brown, S. J., Donath, S., MacArthur, C., McDonald, E. A. and Krastev, A. H. (2010). Urinary incontinence in nulliparous women before and during pregnancy: prevalence, incidence, and associated risk factors. *Int Urogynecol J*, *21*(2), 193-202.

[3]   Martínez Franco, E., Parés, D., Lorente Colomé, N., Méndez Paredes, J. R. and Amat Tardiu, L. (2014). Urinary incontinence during pregnancy. Is there a difference between first and third trimester? *Eur J Obstet Gynecol Reprod Biol*, *182*, 86-90.

[4]   Hvidman, L., Foldspang, A., Mommsen, S. and Nielsen, J. B. (2003). Postpartum urinary incontinence. *Acta Obstet Gynecol Scand*, *82*(6), 556-63.

[5]   MacArthur, C. 1., Wilson, D. 2., Herbison, P., et al. (2016). Urinary incontinence persisting after childbirth: extent, delivery history, and effects in a 12-year longitudinal cohort study. *Br J Obstet Gynaecol*, *123*(6), 1022-9.

[6]   Liebergall-Wischnitzer, M., Cnaan, T., Hochner, H. and Paltiel, O. (2015). Self-reported Prevalence of and Knowledge About Urinary Incontinence Among Community-Dwelling Israeli Women of Child-Bearing Age. *Wound Ostomy Continence Nurs*, *42*(4), 401-6.

[7]   Rincón Ardila, O. (2015). Prevalence and risk factors for urinary incontinence among women consulting in primary care. *Rev Med Chil*, *143*(2), 203-12.

[8]   Virtuoso, J. F., Menezes, E. C. and Mazo. G. Z. (2015). Risk factors for urinary inconti-nence in elderly women practicing physical exercises. *Rev Bras Ginecol Obstet*, *37*(2), 82-6.

[9]   Kaşıkçı, M., Kılıç, D., Avşar, G. and Şirin, M. (2015). Prevalence of urinary incontinence in older Turkish women, risk factors, and effect on activities of daily living. *Arch Gerontol Geriatr*, *61*(2), 217-23.

[10]   Kumari, S. 1., Singh, A. J. and Jain, V. (2008). Treatment seeking behavior for urinary incontinence among north Indian women. *Indian J Med Sci*, *62*(9), 352-6.

[11]   Perera, J., Kirthinanda, D. S., Wijeratne, S. and Wickramarachchi, T. K. (2014). Descriptive cross sectional study on prevalence, perceptions, predisposing factors and health seeking behaviour of women with stress urinary incontinence. *BMC Women's Health*, *14*, 78.

[12]   Robinson, M. and Humpage, C. (2016). Factors affecting help-seeking behaviour of women with urinary incontinence; a commentary providing insights for osteopaths. *Int J Osteopath Med*, doi: 10.1016/ j.ijosm.2016.04.005.

[13]   Koch, L. H. (2006). Help-seeking behaviors of women with urinary incontinence: an integrative literature review. *J Midwifery Womens Health*, *51*(6), 39-44.

[14]   Elbiss, H. M., Osman, N. and Hammad, F. T. (2013). Social impact and healthcare-seeking behavior among women with urinary incontinence in the United Arab Emirates. *Int J Gynaecol Obste*, *122*(2), 136-9.

[15]   Ng, S. F., Lok, M. K., Pang, S. M. and Wun, Y. T. (2014). Stress urinary incontinence in younger women in primary care: prevalence and opportunistic intervention. *J Women Health*, *23*(1), 65-8.

[16]   Hunskaar, S., Burgio, K., Ciark, A., et al. (2005). Epidemiology of Urinary (UI) and Faecal (FI) Incontinence and Pelvic Organ Prolapse (POP). *WHO-ICS International Consultation on Incontinence*. 3rd ed. Paris: Health Publications Ltd.

[17]   Shumaker, S. A., Wyman, J. F, Uebersax, J. S., McClish, D. and Fantl, J. A. (1994). Health-related quality of life measures for women with urinary incontinence: the Incontinence Impact Questionnaire and the Urogenital Distress Inventory. Continence Program in Women (CPW) Research Group. *Qual Life Res*, *3*(5), 291–306.

[18]   Lauver, D., Gross, J., Ruff, C. and Wells, T. (2004). Patient-centered interventions: implications for incontinence. *Nurs Res*, *53*(6S), S30-S35.

[19]   Broome, B. A. (2003). The impact of urinary incontinence on self-efficacy and quality of life. *Health Qual Life Outcomes*, *1*, 35.

[20] Monz, B., Pons, M. E., Hampel, C., et al. (2005). Patient-reported impact of urinary incontinence-results from treatment seeking women in 14 European countries. Maturitas, 52 Suppl 2, 24-34.

[21] Saleh, N., Bener, A., Khenyab, N., Al-Mansori, Z. and Al Muraikhi, A. (2005). Prevalence, awareness and determinants of health care-seeking behaviour for urinary incontinence in Qatari women: a neglected problem? *Maturitas*, *50*(1), 58-65.

[22] Bradway, C., Coyne, K. S., Irwin, D. and Kopp, Z. (2008). Lower urinary tract symptoms in women-a common but neglected problem. *J Am Acad Nurse Pract*, *20*(6), 311-8.

[23] Hägglund, D. and Wadensten, B. (2008). Fear of humiliation inhibits women's care-seeking behaviour for long-term urinary incontinence. *Scand J Caring Sci*, *21*(3), 305-12.

[24] Gasquet, I., Tcherny-Lessenot, S. and Gaudebout, P. (2006). Influence of the severity of stress urinary incontinence on quality of life, health care seeking, and treatment: A national cross-sectional survey. *Eur Urol*, *50*(4), 818-25.

[25] Altintas, R., Beytur, A. and Oguz, F. (2013). Assessment of urinary incontinence in the women in eastern Turkey. *Int Urogynecol J*, *24*(11), 1977-82.

[26] Shaw, C., Das Gupta, R., Williams, K. S., Assassa, R. P. and McGrother, C. (2006). A survey of help-seeking and treatment provision in women with stress urinary incontinence. *BJU Int*, *97*(4), 752-7.

[27] Cooper, J., Annappa, M., Quigley, A., Dracocardos, D., Bondili, A. and Mallen, C. (2015). Prevalence of female urinary incontinence and its impact on quality of life in a cluster population in the United Kingdom (UK): a community survey. *Prim Health Care Res Dev*, *16*(4), 377-82.

[28] Hannestad, Y. S., Rortveit, G. and Hunskaar, S. (2002). Help-seeking and associated factors in female urinary incontinence. The Norwegian EPINCONT Study. Epidemiology of Incontinence in the County of Nord-Trøndelag. *Scand J Prim Health Care*, *20*(2), 102-7.

[29] O'Connell, B, Wellman, D., Baker, L. and Day, K. (2006). Does a continence educational brochure promote health-seeking behavior? *J Wound Ostomy Continence Nurs*, *33*(4), 389-95.

[30] Ruiz de Viñaspre Hernández, R., Tomás Aznar, C. and Rubio Aranda, E. (2014). Factors associated with treatment-seeking behavior for postpartum urinary incontinence. *J Nurs Scholarsh*, *46*(6), 391-7.

[31] Harris, S. S., Link, C. L., Tennstedt, S. L., Kusek, J. W. and McKinlay, J. B. (2007). Care seeking and treatment for urinary incontinence in a diverse population. *J Urol*, *177*(2), 680-4.

[32] Visser, E., de Bock, G. H., Kollen, B. J., Meijerink, M., Berger, M. Y. and Dekker, J. H. (2012). Systematic screening for urinary incontinence in older women: who could benefit from it? *Scand J Prim Health Care*, *30*(1), 21-8.

[33] Cetinel, B., Demirkesen, O. and Tarcan, T. (2007). Hidden female urinary incontinence in urology and obstetrics and gynecology outpatient clinics in Turkey: what are the determi-nants of bothersome urinary incontinence and help-seeking behavior? *Int Urogynecol J Pelvic Floor Dysfunct*, *18*(6), 659-64.

[34] da Silva, L. and Lopes, M. H. (2009). Urinary incontinence in women: reasons for not seeking treatment. *Rev Esc Enferm USP*, *43*(1), 72-8.

[35] El-Azab, A. S. and Shaaban, O. M. (2010). Measuring the barriers against seeking cónsul-tation for urinary incontinence among Middle Eastern women. *BMC Womens Health*, *10*, 3.

[36] Margalith, I., Gillon, G. and Gordon, D. (2004). Urinary incontinence in women under 65: quality of life, stress related to incontinence and patterns of seeking health care. *Qual Life Res*, *13*(8), 1381-90.

[37] Norton, P., MacDonald, L., Sedgwick, P. and Stanton, S. (1988). Distress and delay associated with urinary incontinence, frequency, and urgency in women. *BMJ*, *297*, 1187- 9.

[38] Wang, C., Li, J., Wan, X., Wang, X., Kane, R. L. and Wang, K. (2015). Effects of stigma on Chinese women's attitudes towards seeking treatment for urinary incontinence. *J Clin Nurs*, *24*(7-8), 1112-21.

[39] Bartoli, S., Aguzzi, G. and Tarricone, R. (2010). Impact on quality of life of urinary incontinence and overactive bladder: a systematic literature review. *Urology*, *75*(3), 491-500.

[40] Mason, L., Glen, S., Walton, I. and Hughes, C. (2001). Women's reluctance to seek help for stress incontinence during pregnancy and following childbirth. *Midwifery*, *17*, 212-21.

[41] Taylor, D. W., Weir, M, Cahill, J. J. and Rizk, D. E. (2010). The self-reported prevalence and knowledge of urinary incontinence and barriers to health care-seeking in a community sample of Canadian women. *Am J Med Sci*, *3*(5), 97-102.

[42] Wu, C., Wang, K. F., Sun, T., Xu, D. J. and Palmer, M. H. (2015). Predicting helpseeking intention of women with urinary incontinence in

Jinan, China: a theory of planned behavior model. *J Clin Nur*, *24*(3-4), 457-64.

[43]   Wang, C., Wan, X., Wang, K., Li, J. J., Sun, T. and Guan, X. (2014). Disease stigma and intentions to seek care for stress urinary incontinence among community-dwelling women. *Maturitas*, *77*(4), 351-5.

[44]   Gjerde, J. L., Rortveit, G., Muleta, M. and Blystad, A. (2013). Silently waiting to heal. *Int Urogynecol J*, *24*(6), 953-8.

[45]   Wu, C., Sun, T., Guan, X. and Wang, K. (2015). Predicting delay to treatment of urinary incontinence among urban community-dwelling women in China. *Int J Nurs Sci*, *2*(1), 34–38.

[46]   Dugan, E., Roberts, C. P., Cohen, S. J., Preisser, J. S., Davis, C. C. and Bland, D. R. (2001). Why older community-dwelling adults do not discuss urinary incontinence with their primary care physicians. *J Am Geriatr Soc*, *49*, 462-5.

[47]   Kwon, C. S. and Lee, J. H. (2014). Prevalence, Risk Factors, Quality of Life, and Health-Care Seeking Behaviors of Female Urinary Incontinence: Results From the 4th Korean National Health and Nutrition Examination Survey VI (2007-2009). *Int Neurourol J*, *18*(1), 31-6.

[48]   Rios, A. A., Cardoso, J. R., Rodrigues, M. A. and de Almeida, S. H. (2011). The help-seeking by women with urinary incontinence in Brazil. *Int Urogynecol J*, *22*(7), 879-84.

[49]   Minassian, V. A., Yan, X., Lichtenfeld, M. J., Sun, H. and Stewart, W. F. (2012). The Iceberg of Health Care Utilization in Women with Urinary incontinence. *Int Urogynecol J*, *23*(8), 1087–93.

[50]   Xu, D., Wang, X., Li, J. and Wang, K. (2015). The mediating effect of 'bothersome' urinary incontinence on help seeking intentions among community-dwelling women. *J Adv Nurs*, *71*(2), 315-25.

[51]   Siddiqui, N. Y., Levin, P. J., Phadtare, A., Pietrobon, R. and Ammarell, N. (2014). Perceptions about female urinary incontinence: a systematic review. *Int Urogynecol J*, *25*(7), 863-71.

[52]   Berger, M. B., Patel, D. A., Miller, J. M., Delancey, J. O. and Fenner, D. E. (2011). Racial differences in self-reported healthcare seeking and treatment for urinary incontinence in community-dwelling women from the EPI Study. *Neurourol Urodyn*, *30*(8), 1442-7.

[53]   El-Azab, A. S. and Mascha, E. J. (2015). Arabic validation of the Urogenital Distress Inventory and Adapted Incontinence Impact Questionnaires–short forms. *Neurourol Urodyn*, *28*(1), 33-39.

[54] El-Safty, M. (2004). Women in Egypt: Islamic rights vs. cultural practices. *Sex roles J Res*, *51*, 273-281.

[55] Mohamed, S. A., Kamel, M. A., Shaaban, O. M. and Salem, H. T. (2003). Acceptability for the use of postpartum intrauterine contraceptive devices: Assiut experience. *Med Princ Pract*, *12*(3), 170-175.

[56] O'Donnell, M., Lose, G., Sykes, D., Voss, S. and Hunskaar, S. (2005). Help-seeking behavior and associated factors among women with urinary incontinence in France, Germany, Spain and the United Kingdom. *Eur Urol*, *47*(3), 385-392.

[57] Kinchen, K., Burgio, K., Diokno, A., Fultz, N., Bump, R. and Obenchain, R. (2003). Factors associated with women's decisions to seek treatment for urinary incontinence. *J Women Health*, *12*(7), 687-697.

[58] Yu, H. J. 1., Wong, W. Y. Chen, J. and Chie, W. C. (2003). Quality of life impact and treatment seeking of Chinese women with urinary incontinence. *Qual Life Res*, *12*(3), 327-33.

[59] Dunivan, G. C., Komesu, Y. M., Cichowski, S. B., Lowery, C., Anger, J. T. and Rogers, R. G. (2015). Elder American Indian women's knowledge of pelvic floor disorders and barriers to seeking care. *Female Pelvic Med Reconstr Surg*, *21*(1), 34-8.

[60] Hsieh, C. H., Su, T. H., Chang, S. T., Lin, S. H., Lee, M. C. and Lee, M. Y. (2008). Prevalence of and attitude toward urinary incontinence in postmenopausal women. *Int J Gynaecol Obstet*, *100*, 171–4.

[61] Weiss, M. G., Ramakrishna, J. and Somma, D. (2006). Health-related stigma: rethinking concepts and interventions. *Psychol Health Med*, *11*, 277–87.

[62] Corrigan, P. and Watson, A. C. (2002). The paradox of self-stigma and mental illness. *Clin Psychol*, *9*, 35–53.

[63] Wan, X., Wang, C., Xu, D., Guan, X., Sun, T. and Wang, K. (2014). Disease stigma and its mediating effect on the relationship between symptom severity and quality of life among community-dwelling women with stress urinary incontinence: a study from a Chinese city. *J Clin Nurs*, *23*, 2170-9.

[64] Porrett, T. and Cox, C. (2008). Coping mechanisms in women living with pelvic floor dysfunction. *Gastrointest Nurs*, *6*(3), 30-39.

[65] MacKay, K. and Hemmett, L. (2001). Needs assessment of women with urinary incontinence in a district health authority. *Br J Gen Pract*, *51*(471), 801–4.

[66] Peters, T. J., Horrocks, S., Stoddart, H. and Somerset, M. (2004). Factors associated with variations in older people's use of community-based continence services. *Health Soc Care Community*, *12*(1), 53–62.

[67] Roe, B., Doll, H. and Wilson, K. (1999). Help seeking behaviour and health and social services utilisation by people suffering from urinary incontinence. *Int J Nurs Stud*, *36*(3), 245–253.

[68] Holst, K. and Wilson, P. D. (1988). The prevalence of female urinary incontinence and reasons for not seeking treatment. *N Z Med J*, *101*, 756–758.

[69] Foldspang, A., Mommsen, S., Lam, G. W. and Elving, L. (1922). Parity as a correlate of adult female urinary incontinence prevalence. *J Epidemiol Community Health*, *46*, 595–600.

[70] Adedokun, B. O., Morhason-Bello, I. O., Ojengbede, O. A., Okonkwo, N. S. and Kolade C. (2012). Help-seeking behavior among women currently leaking urine in Nigeria: is it any different from the rest of the world? *Patient Prefer Adherence*, *6*, 815-9.

[71] Shaw, C. 1., Tansey, R., Jackson, C., Hyde, C. and Allan, R. (2001). Barriers to help seeking in people with urinary symptoms. *Fam Pract*, *18*(1), 48-52.

[72] Shaw, C., Gupta, R. D., Bushnell, D. M., et al. (2006). The extent and severity of urinary incontinence amongst women in UK GP waiting rooms. *Fam Pract*, *23*(5), 497–506.

[73] Horrocks, S., Somerset, M., Stoddart, H. and Peters, T. J. (2004). What prevents older people from seeking treatment for urinary incontinence? A qualitative exploration of barriers to the use of community continence services. *Fam Pract*, *21*(6), 689–96.

[74] Basra, R., Cortes, E., Khullar, V. and Kelleher, C. (2009). Do colour and personality influence treatment seeking behaviour in women with lower urinary tract symptoms? A prospective study using the short Luscher colour test. *J Obstet Gynaecol*, *29*(5), 407–11.

[75] Irwin, D. E., Milsom, I., Kopp, Z., Abrams, P. and EPIC Study Group. (2008). Symptom bother and health care-seeking behavior among individuals with overactive bladder. *Eur Urol*, *53*(5), 1029–37

[76] Mitteness, L. S. (1990). Knowledge and beliefs about urinary incontinence in adulthood and old age. *J Am Geriatr Soc*, *38*, 374–378.

[77] Rekers, H., Drogendijk, A. C., Valkenburg, H. and Riphagen, F. (1992). Urinary incontinence in women from 35 to 79 years of age: prevalence and consequences. *Eur J Obstet Gynecol Reprod Biol*, *43*, 229–234.

[78] Reymert, J. and Hunskaar, S. (1994). Why do only a minority of perimenopausal women with urinary incontinence consult a doctor? *Scand J Prim Health Care*, *12*, 180–183.

[79] Hemachandra, N. N., Rajapaksa, L. C. and Manderson, L. (2009). A "usual occurrence": stress incontinence among reproductive aged women in Sri Lanka. *Soc Sci Med*, *69*(9), 1395–1401.

[80] Buurman, M. B. and Lagro-Janssen, A. L. (2013). Women's perception of postpartum pelvic floor dysfunction and their help-seeking behaviour: a qualitative interview study. *Scand J Caring Sci*, *27*(2), 406-13.

[81] Higa, R. and Lopes, M. H. (2007). Why the nursing staff professionals with urinary incontinence do not seek for treatment. *Rev Bras Enferm*, *60*(5), 503-6.

[82] Waetjen, L. E., Xing, G., Johnson, W. O., Melnikow, J., Gold, E. B. and Study of Women's Health Across the Nation (SWAN). (2015). Factors associated with seeking treatment for urinary incontinence during the menopausal transition. *Obstet Gynecol*, *125*(5), 1071-9.

[83] Minassian, V. A., Devore, E., Hagan, K. and Grodstein, F. (2013). Severity of urinary incontinence and effect on quality of life in women by incontinence type. *Obstet Gynecol*, *121*(5), 1083-90.

[84] Teunissen, D., van Weel, C. and Lagro-Janssen, T. (2005). Urinary incontinence in older people living in the community: examining help-seeking behaviour. *Br J Gen Pract*, *55*(519), 776-82.

[85] Hagglund, D., Walker-Engstrom, M., Larsson, G. and Leppert, J. (2003). Reasons why women with long-term urinary incontinence do not seek professional help: A cross-sectional population-based cohort study. *Int Urogynecol J*, *14*, 296- 304.

[86] Kirss, F., Lang, K., Toompere, K. and Veerus, P. (2013). Prevalence and risk factors of urinary incontinence among Estonian postmenopausal women. *Springerplus*, *2*, 524.

[87] Shaw, C. (2001). A review of the psychosocial predictors of help-seeking behaviour and impact on quality of life in people with urinary incontinence. *J Clin Nurs*, *10*, 15-24.

[88] Wagg, A. and Bunn, F. (2007). Unassisted pelvic floor exercises for postnatal women: a systematic review. *J Adv Nurs*, *58*(5), 407-417.

[89] Goldstein, M., Hawthorne, M. E., Engeberg, S., McDowell, B. J. and Burgio, K. L. (1992). Urinary incontinence. Why people do not seek help. *J Gerontol Nurs*, *18*(4), 15-20.

[90] Dumoulin, C. and Hay-Smith, J. (2010). Pelvic floor muscle training versus no treatment, or inactive control treatments, for urinary incontinence in women. *Cochrane Database Syst Rev*, (1), CD005654.

[91] Wan, X. J., Li, J. J., Wang, X. J., et al. (2014). The bothersomeness of female urinary incontinence and its influencing factors: study from a Chinese city. *Int J Nurs Sci*, *1*, 58-63.

[92] St. John, W., Griffiths, S., Wallis, M. and McKenzie, S. (2013). Women's management of urinary incontinence in daily living. *J Wound Ostomy Continence Nurs*, *40*(5), 524–532.

[93] Papanicolaou, S., Pons, M. E., Hampel, C., et al. (2005). Medical resource utilisation and cost of care for women seeking treatment for urinary incontinence in an outpatient setting. Examples from three countries participating in the PURE study. *Maturitas*, *52* Suppl 2, S35-47.

[94] Fritel, X., Panjo, H., Varnoux, N. and Ringa, V. (2014). The individual determinants of care-seeking among middle-aged women reporting urinary incontinence: analysis of a 2273-woman cohort. *Neurourol Urodyn*, *33*(7), 1116-22.

[95] Lin, S. Y. and Dougherty, M. C. (2003). Incontinence impact, symptom distress and treatment-seeking behavior in women with involuntary urine loss in Southern Taiwan. *Int J Nurs Stud*, *40*(3), 227-34.

[96] Sexton, C. C., Coyne, K. S., Kopp, Z. S., et al., (2009). The overlap of storage, voiding and postmicturition symptoms and implications for treatment seeking in the USA, UK and Sweden: EpiLUTS. *BJU Int*, 103 Suppl 3, 12–23.

[97] Andersson, G., Johansson, J. E., Sahlberg-Blom, E., Pettersson, N. and Nilsson K. (2005). Urinary incontinence--why refraining from treatment? A population based study. *Scand J Urol Nephrol*, *39*(4), 301-7.

[98] Howard, F. and Steggall, M. (2010). Urinary incontinence in women: quality of life and help-seeking. *Br J Nurs*, *19*(12), 742, 744, 746, 748-9.

[99] Bradway, C. and Strumpf, N. (2008). Seeking care: women's narratives concerning long-term urinary incontinence. *Urol Nurs*, *28*(2), 123-9.

[100] Melville, J. L., Newton, K., Fan, M. Y. and Katon, W. (2006). Health care discussions and treatment for urinary incontinence in U.S. women. *Am J Obstet Gynecol*, *194*(3), 729-37.

[101] Yip, S. K. and Chung, T. K. (2003). Treatment-seeking behavior in Hong Kong Chinese women with urinary symptoms. *Int Urogynecol J Pelvic Floor Dysfunct*, *14*(1), 27-30.

[102] Sangi-Haghpeykar, H., Mozayeni, P., Young, A. and Fine, P. M. (2008). Stress urinary incontinence and counseling and practice of pelvic floor exercises postpartum in low-income Hispanic women. *Int Urogynecol J Pelvic Floor Dysfunct*, *19*(3), 361-365.

[103] Hermansen, I. L., O'Connell, B. and Gaskin, C. J. (2010). Are postpartum women in denmark being given helpful information about urinary incontinence and pelvic floor exercises? *J Midwifery Womens Health*, *55*(2), 171-174.

[104] Sangsawang, B. and Sangsawang, N. (2015). Prevention and treatment of stress urinary incontinence during pregnancy: global perspective, research to practice In: Dennel G, editor. *Midwifery: global perspectives, practices and challenges*. New York: Nova Science Publishers.

[105] Whitford, H. M., Alder, B. and Jones, M. (2007). A cross-sectional study of knowledge and practice of pelvic floor exercises during pregnancy and associated symptoms of stress urinary incontinence in North-East Scotland. *Midwifery*, *23*(2), 204-217.

[106] Rozensky, R. H., Tovian, S. M., Gartley, C. B., Nichols, T. R. and Layton, M. (2013). A quality of life survey of individuals with urinary incontinence who visit a self-help website: implications for those seeking healthcare information. *J Clin Psychol Med Settings*, *20*(3), 275-83.

[107] Alewijnse, D., Mesters, I., Metsemakers, J., Ad-riaans, J. and van den Borne, B. (2001). Predictors of intention to adhere to physiotherapy among women with urinary incontinence. *Health Ed Res*, *16*, 173-186.

[108] Reducing Spencer, J. (2009). Barriers and improving access to continence care: examining the evidence. *Urol Nurs*, *29*(6), 405-13.

[109] National Institute for Health and Clinical Excellence (2006) Urinary incontinence: the management of urinary incontinence in women. http:// guidance.nice.org.uk/CG40.

[110] Alappattu, M., Neville, C., Beneciuk, J. and Bishop, M. (2016). Urinary incontinence symptoms and impact on quality of life in patients seeking outpatient physical therapy services. *Physiother Theory Pract*, *32*(2), 107-12.

[111] Joanna Briggs Institute. (2006). A pelvic floor muscle exercise programme for urinary incontinence following childbirth. *Nurs Stand*, *20*(33), 46-50.

In: Urinary Incontinence
Editor: Debra Newton

ISBN: 978-1-53610-099-0
© 2016 Nova Science Publishers, Inc.

Chapter 4

ADVANCES IN NON-SURGICAL MANAGEMENT OF URINARY INCONTINENCE

Ran Pang[1,*], Yun-Xiang Xiao[2,3], Lei-Lei Qi[1]
and Jian-Xin Lu[1]
[1]Department of Urology, Guang An Men Hospital,
China Academy of Chinese Medical Sciences, Beijing, China
[2]Department of Urology, Peking University First Hospital,
Beijing, China
[3]Institute of Urology, Peking University,
National Urological Cancer Center, Beijing, China

ABSTRACT

Urinary incontinence (UI) is a common disease in elderly women. It is classified into stress UI, urgency UI and mixed UI based on different etiology. It has been recommended that potential benefits and risks should be considered before a therapeutic strategy being developed for patients with UI. Compared to surgery, non-surgical management is more likely to be accepted by patients. Furthermore, more and more evidences have show the efficacy of these non-invasive treatment. In this chapter, we will present the evidence about the effectiveness of these treatments,

---

[*] Correspondence: Ran Pang, MD, PhD Department of Urology, Guang An Men Hospital, China Academy of Chinese Medical Sciences. No. 5 Bei Xian Ge Street, Xi Cheng District, Beijing, China, 100053, FAX: +8610-63014195, Telephone: +8610-88001040, e-mail: pangran2002@gmail.com or pangran2002@sina.com.

as well as their potential mechanism, on different types of UI. In terms of specific treatment, lifestyle interventions, behavioral and physical therapies, and pharmacological management will be discussed for each type of UI. Besides, the complementary and alternative medicine treatment will also be involved. In particular, we will share our clinical experience and present the evidence from our research in management of UI.

INTRODUCTION

Urinary incontinence (UI) is a common condition in female population. It is estimated that approximate 200 million women are affected by UI worldwide [1]. The reported prevalence of female UI is as high as 55% in the literature [2]. In general, UI is classified into stress urinary incontinence (SUI), urgency urinary incontinence (UUI), mixed urinary incontinence (MUI). With the development of surgical technique, a number of patients with UI can be cured. Nowadays, mid-urethral sling has been a popular treatment for SUI due to its definite efficacy. Besides, sacral nerve stimulation has been used widely for refractory overactive bladder (OAB) and UUI. However, these surgeries are relatively invasive and their short-term and long-term complications are bothersome for patients. Compared to surgery, non-invasive management is more likely to be accepted by patients with UI. Basically, the non-surgical management of UI includes lifestyle interventions, behavioral and physical therapies, pharmacological management, and complementary and alternative medicine (CAM) therapies. In this chapter, the efficacy and safety of each intervention on different types of UI will be presented.

LIFESTYLE INTERVENTION

Women with all types of UI should be advised to change their lifestyle including smoking cessation, weight loss and dietary modification. A case control study showed a strong relationship between cigarette smoking and UI in women. Based on result of this study, the odds radio for SUI and UUI was 2.48 (95% CI 1.60 - 3.84) and 2.92 (95% CI 1.58 - 5.39) for current smoker respectively [3]. Another study further revealed that heavy smokers were more likely to suffer from UUI [4], which might result from irritative effects of cigarette on the detrusor. Additionally, chronic cough caused by smoking could be an important contributor for SUI [5]. According to these findings, smoking cessation is recommended for all patients with UI.

Some studies have demonstrated the relationship between increased body mass index (BMI) and UI. A cross sectional study based on female Saudi population showed that higher BMI was associated with increasing risk of urinary infection and consequently UI [6]. Another study showed that women with higher BMI were more likely to develop UUI and MUI [7]. To assess the effect of weight loss on UI, a number of clinical trials were designed and performed. In a randomized controlled trial (RCT), 338 women with UI were allocated to weight loss group or control group with a 2:1 ratio. After 12 months, patients in weight loss group presented a more significant reduction in weekly SUI episodes compared to the counterparts in control group (65% vs. 47%, P<0.001). After 18 months, a greater proportion of women with more than 70% improvement in UUI episodes was found in weight loss group compared to control group [8]. Anger et al. further found that all UI patients BMI of more than 25 can get benefit from weight loss [9].

Dietary modification is another lifestyle intervention for women with UI. It is reported that some food and beverages may aggravate UI. Of those, caffeinated beverages are considered as the most important contributor for all types of UI. A prospective cohort study demonstrated that excessive caffeine intake (≥450 mg/day) was associated with the development of UI [10]. A case-control study observed the effect of caffeine on bladder based on urodynamic evaluation. The results showed that high caffeine intake (≥400 mg/day) was associated with detrusor overactivity [11]. A cross-sectional, nationally representative survey found that moderate caffeine intake (≥204 mg/day) was the independent risk factor for all types of UI, after controlling other factors [12]. Some studies further found that caffeine reduction regimen might be helpful for UI patients. In an early study, 41 elderly rural women were instructed to reduce caffeine intake by a home-visited nurse. After four weeks, their daily consumption of caffeinated beverages was reduced from 829 ± 385 to 489 ± 312 ml. As a result, their daily urinary leakage and UI episodes were decreased from 42.21 ± 77.34 to 24.09±40.93 and from 2.60 ± 2.65 to 1.68 ± 1.52 respectively [13]. A prospective RCT showed that reduced caffeine intake could improve patients' lower urinary tract symptoms (LUTS) significantly, but had no effect on reduction of urinary leakage [14]. Besides caffeinated beverages, carbonated drinks are another daily consumption which may exacerbate the UI symptoms. A prospective cohort study found that consumption of carbonated drinks was associated with the development of SUI after analyzing data from 7046 women [15]. Another study found that excessive intake of carbonated beverages increased risk to develop UI, but mild and moderate consumption did not [16]. In addition, an survey based on community population showed that some other diets and beverages including spicy foods, citrus juices, and tomato-based products may trigger UI [17].

Management of fluid intake in UI patients remains a big issue. A prospective, randomized, crossover study assessed the effect of increasing and decreasing fluid intake on symptoms in women with urodynamic diagnosed SUI or detrusor overactibvity. The result showed that fluid intake restriction can relieve LUTS and decrease UI episodes for each kind of patients [18]. Another prospective, randomized, crossover study showed that a 25% reduction in fluid intake could improve OAB symptoms significnatly [19].

According to current available evidence, a lifestyle intervention strategy including smoking cessation, weight loss and decrease of fluid intake, caffeine and carbonated drinks is recommended for patients with all types of UI [20].

BEHAVIORAL AND PHYSICAL THERAPIES

Behavioral and physical therapies refer to a series of self-motivated personal retraining and related techniques which can enhance the effect of retraining. These therapies generally include bladder training, pelvic floor muscle training (PFMT), biofeedback and posterior tibial nerve stimulation (PTNS).

Bladder Training

Bladder training refers to a self-control technique performed by patients, which is used to relieve the symptoms of UI. Timed voiding is the most common technique for patients to practice bladder training. Typically, patients need to complete a three-day bladder diary to present their current voiding habit. Then an individual voiding schedule can be published by adding 15 minutes to the current voiding interval. Patients are asked to void according to the schedule strictly, no matter whether they actually feel the urge to void or not. Once they are accustomed to the schedule, the interval between two micturitions will be increased gradually, until they can last for three hours without feeling urge to void. Traditionally, bladder training is considered as an effective approach for OAB and UUI. Some studies further assessed the effect of bladder training on other types of UI. In an early study, 88 women with SUI and 35 women with UUI were managed by bladder training. After treatment, the overall episodes of UI and urine leakage were reduced by 57% and 54% respectively and no difference was found between two groups, which revealed that bladder training is effective for both SUI and UUI [21]. A systematic review has also confirmed the effectiveness of bladder training on UUI, SUI and MUI [22]. In order to achieve certain effect, bladder training should be practiced for a minimum of 6 weeks. Importantly, patients may experience some minor discomfort during the treatment. To ensure that patients can complete 6-week treatment, it is highly recommended to communicate with patients prior to the treatment.

PFMT

PFMT is another self-control technique designed to strengthen the muscles of pelvic floor. With the enhancement of pelvic floor function, SUI can be improved significantly. Furthermore, PFMT can inhibit detrusor overactivity in patients with OAB [23], which may contribute to the improvement of UUI. A RCT showed that 12-week PFMT can reduce the urine leakage evaluated by 1-hour pad test (5.1 g vs. 1.5 g, $P<0.01$) and increase the pelvic floor muscle strength significantly in patients with SUI or MUI [24]. A systematic review published in Cochrane collaboration has further confirmed the effect of PFMT on each type of UI. That review also showed that PFMT had less efficacy in patients with MUI in comparison with ones with pure SUI [25]. To obtain substantial benefit, PFMT should normally be lasted for at least 8 to 12 weeks. Once patients get benefit from this exercise, PFMT is recommended to be performed for a longer time to maintain its effect. The majority of patients with UI, however, fail to practice a long-term PFMT. A follow-up study revealed that only 41.6% of women with SUI adhered to PFMT for five years [26]. Another study demonstrated that the rate of adherence was only 28% in patients with SUI during the 15 years follow-up period [27]. A study compared the effects of PFMT and bladder training on SUI in elderly women. The result showed that PFMT is more effective than bladder training in management of SUI [28].

Biofeedback

Biofeedback refers to a modern technique to instruct patients to perform the right PFMT. Traditionally, it is believed that the efficacy of biofeedback relies on the effect of PFMT. An RCT showed that biofeedback had similar effectiveness with PFMT in women with SUI [29]. However, an systematic review showed that biofeedback could provide an add-on effect to PFMT for women with any type of UI [30]. Another study further revealed that detrusor overactivity was a risk factor for patients to fail to biofeedback [31]. Based on our experience, women with pure SUI seem to obtain more benefit from biofeedback compared to ones with UUI or MUI.

PTNS

PTNS is typically performed by a small needle which is inserted above the medial aspect of the ankle and connected to an electrical stimulator. Electrical stimulation of the posterior tibial nerve transmits the signal to sacral micturition center through S2-S4 sacral nerve plexus, which can modulate lower urinary tract function effectively. To obtain the substantial effect, all patients are recommended to complete 12 weekly treatment of 30 minutes each. A multicenter RCT compared the efficacy of PTNS and tolterodine for OAB. In it, 100 patients with OAB were allocated to receiving weekly PTNS or 4mg daily tolterodine for 12 weeks. After treatment, 79.5% of patients in PTNS group reported a significant improvement compared to 54.8% in tolterodine group (p = 0.01) [32]. To evaluate the long-term effectiveness of PTNS, the same authors provided an additional 9 months of treatment for the patients with good response to PTNS. During 12 months follow-up, the daily episodes of UI and moderate to severe urgency were decreased by 1.6 and 3.7 respectively [33]. In a multicenter double-blinded RCT, sham treatment was used as control. Based on the result of this study, a significant higher proportion in patients with a satisfactory improvement was found in PTNS group compared to sham group (54.5 vs. 20.9, P<0.01) [34]. A systematic review further presented that the success rates of PTNS for idiopathic OAB varied from 54% to 93% [35].

Some studies focus on the efficacy of PTNS on neurogenic OAB. Kabay et al. treated 19 patients with neurogenic OAB secondary to multiple sclerosis. They found that 12 -week PTNS could not only improve the symptoms but also increase patients' mean volume at the first involuntary detrusor contraction and mean maximum cystometric capacity [36]. Five years later, same authors reported the long-term effect of PTNS on neurogenic OAB in 34 patients with multiple sclerosis. They found that 12 months PTNS could decrease the daily episodes of UI and urgency by 3.4 and 7.4 respectively [37]. Recently, they further presented the effectiveness of PTNS for OAB secondary to Parkinson's disease. In that study, 47 patients received 12 weeks PTNS. After treatment, patients' daily UUI and urgency episodes were reduced by 3.1 and 6.3 respectively. By contrast, the mean first involuntary detrusor contraction volume was increased from 133.2 ± 48.1 to 237.3 ± 43.1 ml, so did the mean maximum cystometric capacity (202.2 ± 36.5 vs. 292.1 ± 50.6 ml) [38].

Pharmacological Management

Pharmacological treatment is a therapeutic option for UI patients who do not have response to behavioral and physical therapies. The medications for OAB and UUI mainly consist of antimuscarinic drugs and beta-3 adrenergic receptor agonist, which have gotten the approval from the US Food and Drug Administration. By contrast, there is no drug approved for the treatment of SUI so far. Some drugs are tired to treat SUI off-label. Of those, duloxetine presents a certain effectiveness for SUI based on current evidence.

Antimuscarinic Drugs

Antimuscarinic drugs have been considered as the mainstay of treatment for OAB and UUI. The current available agents includes oxybutynin, tolterodine, solifenacin, fesoterodine, darifenacin, trospium, and propiverine. A number of studies have shown their efficacy and safety for the treatment of OAB and UUI. A systematic review confirmed that antimuscarinic drugs were more effective than placebo in treatment of OAB. However, a significant more adverse events were observed in patients taking antimuscarinic drugs compared to ones on placebo (29.6% vs. 7.9%) [39]. Another systematic review demonstrated that antimuscarinic drugs monotherapy or combined with bladder training were superior to bladder training alone for patients with OAB [40]. To optimize antimuscarinic therapy for OAB, Buser et al. performed two network meta-analyses to quantity the efficacy and safety across different drugs, dosages, and pharmaceutical forms. They found that trospium chloride (40 mg/d), oxybutynin topical gel (100mg/g per day), and fesoterodine (4 mg/d) seemed to have the best efficacy, while higher dosages of orally administered oxybutynin and propiverine were more intolerable in patients with OAB [41]. The common adverse events of antimuscarinic drugs includes dry mouth, constipation, urinary retention, and blurred vision. In addition, it is reported that antimuscarinic drugs may cause the cognitive dysfunction in elderly patients. A prospective cohort study showed that 23.2% of elderly patients taking antimuscarinic drugs developed dementia during a mean follow-up of 7.3 years [42]. In terms of specific agents, oxybutynin is more likely to cause cognitive dysfunction, because it can cross the blood-brain barrier and bind to type-1 muscarinic receptor located in the brain, which may result in the disorder of central nervous system [43]. Compared to oxybutynin, trospium has more safety for elderly patients because it cannot penetrate the blood-brain barrier [43].

Beta-3 Adrenergic Receptor Agonist

Mirabegron is the first clinically available beta-3 adrenergic receptor agonist, which has been used for treatment of OAB and UUI. It has been affirmed that beta-3 adrenergic receptor has a predominant expression in detrusor and its activation can induce detrusor relaxation. On one hand, mirabegron can active beta-3 adrenergic receptor and consequently mediate the detrusor relaxation through cyclic adenosine monophosphate pathway [44]. On the other hand, mirabegron can reduce the amount of acetylcholine by acting on the cholinergic pathway, which also contributes to the detrusor relaxation [45]. A prospective, double-blind, placebo-controlled RCT showed that mirabegron was superior to placebo significantly in improvement of OAB and UUI symptoms. Daily 50 mg and 100mg mirabegron could reduce daily episodes of UI by 1.5 and 1.6 respectively [46]. A systematic review showed that mirabegron at daily dosages of 25 mg, 50 mg, and 100mg could reduce the episodes of UI and urgency significantly. Furthermore, 50 mg and 100mg mirabegron could improve OAB symptoms as early as four weeks after treatment [47]. Chapple et al. pooled data from three phase 3 RCTs and performed a post hoc analysis. They found that daily 50 mg mirabegron was effective for OAB and its effect seemed to be enhanced with an increase in severity of UI [48]. Compared to antimuscarinic drugs, the adverse events of mirabegron is rare. The reported side effects include hypertension, nasopharyngitis and urinary tract infection.

Duloxetine

Duloxetine is a reuptake inhibitor of serotonin and norepinephrine, which is used for treatment of SUI in the UK. It is reported that duloxetinecan can increase the concentration of serotonin and norepinephrine in the sacral spinal cord, and consequently enhance the resting tone and contraction strength of the urethral sphincter. In a multicenter placebo-controlled RCT, 2758 women with SUI were allocated to receiving daily 80 mg duloxetine or placebo. After 6-week treatment, weekly episodes of UI were decreased by 50% in duloxetine group, which was significant greater than 29.9% in placebo group. Moreover, patients in duloxetine group presented a more significant improvement in weekly pad use compared to counterparts in placebo group (31.4% vs. 12.5%) [49]. The subsequent open-label extension study showed that the efficacy of duloxetine was maintained over 72 weeks [49]. Two other open-label studies with a follow-up of more than one year affirmed the long-term efficacy of duloxetine for SUI [50, 51]. A systematic review showed that 52.5% of patients taking duloxetine presented an improvement of more than 50% in daily episodes of UI, compared to 33.7% of patients receiving placebo [52]. A placebo-controlled RCT further assessed the effect of duloxetine on OAB and UUI. The results revealed that 12-week treatment of duloxetine (daily 80 mg for 4 weeks and subsequently increased to daily 120 mg for 8 weeks) could improve the OAB symptoms and decrease the episodes of UI and urgency [53]. The reported adverse events was as high as 62.7%, including dry mouth, nausea, constipation, and fatigue, which results in a high rate of treatment discontinuation.

CAM Therapies

CAM refers to a series of medical and health care practices and products that are not considered to be part of conventional medicine [54]. The National Center for Complementary and Alternative Medicine at the NIH has grouped CAM into five domains: (1) biologically-based therapies, such as nutraceuticals; (2) mind-body interventions, such as yoga; (3) manipulative and body-based approaches, such as massage; (4) energy therapies, such as Qigong and Reiki; (5) whole medical systems, such as acupuncture [55].

Acupuncture
Acupuncture, as an important component of traditional Chinese medicine, has gained acceptance in urologists over the past decades [56]. A number of studies have shown its effect on each type of UI. However, it remains a challenge to develop a perfect control intervention in acupuncture trials. To minimize the bias, Liu et al. created a new pragmatic placebo needle with a blunt tip. In order to perform the placebo intervention, a small pad is adhered to patients' skin of each acupoint and placebo needle only pierce the pad without penetrating the skin. A study has demonstrated that the placebo needle is able to blind patients effectively [57]. Based on the instrument, a series of single-blind RCTs were designed to assess the effect of acupuncture on SUI. In phase I study, 70 patients with SUI were assigned to receive electro-acupuncture or placebo acupuncture acting on bilateral BL33 and BL35 for six weeks. After treatment, patients in electro-acupuncture group presented a more significant decrease in the urine leakage and episodes of SUI than the

counterparts in control group (2.3 vs. 0.3 g, and 2.0 vs. 0.7) [58]. To observe the long-term efficacy of acupuncture, a single-center RCT was carried out. In it, 80 patients with SUI received real or placebo electro-acupuncture for six weeks and subsequently were followed 24 weeks. During the follow-up period, the median 72-hour episodes of SUI were reduced by 3.25 in electro-acupuncture group, which was greater than 1.0 in control group. Besides, a more significant improvement in International Consultation on Incontinence Questionnaire-Short Form (ICIQ-SF) score was also observed in electro-acupuncture group compared to control group [59]. In addition, a multi-centered, phase II RCT is ongoing, which may provide strong evidence for the long-term effectiveness of acupuncture on management of SUI [60].

Some studies observed the efficacy of acupuncture for treatment of UUI. In a single-blind RCT, 50 patients with OAB refractory to antimuscarinics were allocated to receiving real or sham electro-acupuncture for six weeks. In electro-acupuncture group, needles were inserted into bilateral BL32, BL33 and BL34 and each pair of needles were connected to the electrodes of electro-acupuncture device, with a disperse-dense (4/20hz) wave for 30 minutes, 5 sessions a week. In control group, non-acupoints with superficial needles were used as sham intervention. To minimize the bias in assessment, the effectiveness of acupuncture was evaluated by urodynamic examination in the study. After treatment, patients in electro-acupuncture group presented a more significant improvement in first sensation of bladder filling, first urge to void and maximum cystometric capacity in comparison with controls [61]. Another RCT assessed the effect of complex acupuncture intervention on UUI. Based on the study protocol, 199 patients with UUI were assigned into electro-acupuncture or tolterodine group with a ratio of 2:1. In terms of acupuncture procedure, two groups of acupoints were used for acupuncture intervention alternately. One included CV3, bilateral KI12, ST28 and SP6 and the other included bilateral BL32, BL35, BL29 and BL40. Of those, two pairs of acupoints (KI12 and ST28; BL32 and BL35) were used to perform electro-acupuncture. After 3-week treatment, the ICIQ-SF score in electro-acupuncture group dropped from 4.06 ± 1.36 to 1.57 ± 1.14 (P<0.01), while no significant difference was found in tolterodine group [62].

MUI is a coexistence of SUI and UUI, which is more bothersome and has greater negative effect on quality of life than SUI and UUI [63]. It is reported that patients with MUI normally respond poorly to both pharmacological and surgical treatment [64]. We designed a series of studies to observe the effect of acupuncture on MUI. In a pilot study, we treated 42 women with MUI using acupuncture for 8 weeks. The acupoints include bilateral BL32, BL35, SP6, and ST36. Of those, BL32 and BL35 were selected for electro-acupuncture therapy. After treatment, the majority of patients presented a significant decrease in ICIQ-SF score and daily episodes of UI, so did the daily urine leakage [65]. To assess the synergy effect of acupuncture and antimuscarinics on MUI, a RCT was designed and carried out. In it, 71 patients with MUI were allocated to receive acupuncture monotherapy or acupuncture combined with daily 4mg tolterodine for 8 weeks. The specific acupuncture procedure was same as the one in pilot study. After treatment, a more significant improvement in daily urine leakage was observed in combination therapy group compared to the control group, while no marked difference was found between two groups in terms of the cured and response rate [66]. To further explore the synergy effect of acupuncture and Chinese herbal therapy, we designed another RCT, which has not recruited the participants yet. In this study, patients with MUI will be assigned to acupuncture, Chinese herbal therapy, combination therapy or placebo group. We hope this study can provide stronger evidence for the efficacy of acupuncture.

Massage

It is reported that massage can relax pelvic floor muscle and regulate the function of center nerve system [67], which may be helpful for patients to relieve LUTS. Kassolik et al. reported a successful case that a 50-year-old woman with SUI was treated by massage. Following four weeks treatment, the patient achieved an 100% improvement in her symptoms of UI [68]. Although only limited evidence is available, we find that massage is effective for each type of UI. The specific efficacy of massage on UI is needed to be verified in well-designed RCT.

Yoga

Some studies have shown that Yoga can improve LUTS effectively in patients with UI, which may result from its modulation for pelvic floor muscle tone [69]. A study showed that Yoga could relieve the symptoms of UUI and improve patients' quality of life [70]. In a RCT, 19 women with UI were allocated to Yoga therapy or control group. After 6-week therapy, women in Yoga therapy group presented a more significant decrease in daily episodes of UI than counterparts in control group (1.8 vs. 0.3) [71]. In terms of specific yoga postures, frog pose, fish pose, locust pose, plank pose, sitting forward bend and seated twist are reported to be beneficial for UI [69].

Energy Therapies

Energy therapies have been considered as a good approach for people to maintain their health. Although the exact mechanism is still not clear, energy therapies have been used for treatment of some chronic diseases including UI. A retrospective study observed the effect of extracorporeal magnetic energy stimulation on SUI and OAB. A total of 72 patients completed a 9-week therapy of magnetic energy stimulation. After treatment, the majority of patients achieved a significant improvement in their symptoms [72]. Qigong is an important form of energy therapies. Unfortunately, no studies focus on its effect on UI so far. We find that Qigong can benefit patients with each types of UI though the effect varies from person to person. Prospective RCTs are needed to provide strong evidence for the efficacy of energy therapies.

SUMMARY

Although the effectiveness of various surgeries for UI, especially SUI, has been widely reported, non-surgical treatment is still considered as the initial management for all types of UI. In terms of specific treatment, lifestyle, behavioral and physical interventions should be the fundamental therapy for all patients with UI. A lot of evidence has shown the efficacy of different medications on UI, but the adverse events should be taken into account prior to using these drugs. In addition, diverse CAM treatments provide more therapeutic options for patients with UI, which allows patients to practice an individualized therapeutic strategy.

ACKNOWLEDGMENT

This work was supported by Beijing Municipal Science and Technology Commission No. Z161100000516156 and grant 2014S292 from Guang An Men Hospital, China Academy of Chinese Medical Sciences. We are also thankful to Dr. Xinyao Zhou for substantial suggestion.

REFERENCES

[1]   Norton, P. and L. Brubaker, Urinary incontinence in women. *Lancet*, 2006. 367(9504): p. 57-67.

[2]   Thom, D., Variation in estimates of urinary incontinence prevalence in the community: effects of differences in definition, population characteristics, and study type. *J. Am. Geriatr. Soc.*, 1998. 46(4): p. 473-80.

[3]   Bump, R.C. and D.K. McClish, Cigarette smoking and urinary incontinence in women. *Am. J. Obstet. Gynecol.*, 1992. 167(5): p. 1213-8.

[4]   Tampakoudis, P., et al., Cigarette smoking and urinary incontinence in women--a new calculative method of estimating the exposure to smoke. *Eur. J. Obstet. Gynecol. Reprod. Biol.*, 1995. 63(1): p. 27-30.

[5]   Fuganti, P.E., J.M. Gowdy, and N.C. Santiago, Obesity and smoking: are they modulators of cough intravesical peak pressure in stress urinary incontinence? *Int. Braz. J. Urol.*, 2011. 37(4): p. 528-33.

[6]   Saadia, Z., Effect of Age, Educational Status, Parity and BMI on Development of Urinary Incontinence - a Cross Sectional Study in Saudi Population. *Mater. Sociomed.*, 2015. 27(4): p. 251-4.

[7]   Townsend, M.K., et al., BMI, waist circumference, and incident urinary incontinence in older women. *Obesity (Silver Spring)*, 2008. 16(4): p. 881-6.

[8]   Wing, R.R., et al., Effect of weight loss on urinary incontinence in overweight and obese women: results at 12 and 18 months. *J. Urol.*, 2010. 184(3): p. 1005-10.

[9]   Anger, J.T., et al., Development of quality indicators for women with urinary incontinence. *Neurourol. Urodyn.*, 2013. 32(8): p. 1058-63.

[10]   Jura, Y.H., et al., Caffeine intake, and the risk of stress, urgency and mixed urinary incontinence. *J. Urol.*, 2011. 185(5): p. 1775-80.

[11]   Arya, L.A., D.L. Myers, and N.D. Jackson, Dietary caffeine intake and the risk for detrusor instability: a case-control study. *Obstet. Gynecol.*, 2000. 96(1): p. 85-9.

[12]   Gleason, J.L., et al., Caffeine and urinary incontinence in US women. *Int. Urogynecol. J.*, 2013. 24(2): p. 295-302.

[13]   Tomlinson, B.U., et al., Dietary caffeine, fluid intake and urinary incontinence in older rural women. *Int. Urogynecol. J. Pelvic Floor Dysfunct.*, 1999. 10(1): p. 22-8.

[14]   Bryant, C.M., C.J. Dowell, and G. Fairbrother, Caffeine reduction

education to improve urinary symptoms. *Br. J. Nurs.*, 2002. 11(8): p. 560-5.

[15] Dallosso, H.M., et al., The association of diet and other lifestyle factors with overactive bladder and stress incontinence: a longitudinal study in women. *BJU Int.*, 2003. 92(1): p. 69-77.

[16] Ozgur Yeniel, A., et al., The prevalence of probable overactive bladder, associated risk factors and its effect on quality of life among Turkish midwifery students. *Eur. J. Obstet. Gynecol. Reprod. Biol.*, 2012. 164(1): p. 105-9.

[17] Thomas, A.M. and J.M. Morse, Managing urinary incontinence with self-care practices. *J. Gerontol. Nurs.*, 1991. 17(6): p. 9-14.

[18] Swithinbank, L., H. Hashim, and P. Abrams, The effect of fluid intake on urinary symptoms in women. *J. Urol.*, 2005. 174(1): p. 187-9.

[19] Hashim, H. and P. Abrams, How should patients with an overactive bladder manipulate their fluid intake? BJU Int, 2008. 102(1): p. 62-6.

[20] Wood, L.N. and J.T. Anger, Urinary incontinence in women. *BMJ*, 2014. 349: p. g4531.

[21] Fantl, J.A., et al., Efficacy of bladder training in older women with urinary incontinence. *JAMA*, 1991. 265(5): p. 609-13.

[22] Wallace, S.A., et al., Bladder training for urinary incontinence in adults. *Cochrane Database Syst. Rev.*, 2004(1): p. CD001308.

[23] Berghmans, B., et al., Efficacy of physical therapeutic modalities in women with proven bladder overactivity. *Eur. Urol.*, 2002. 41(6): p. 581-7.

[24] Celiker Tosun, O., et al., Does pelvic floor muscle training abolish symptoms of urinary incontinence? A randomized controlled trial. *Clin. Rehabil.*, 2015. 29(6): p. 525-37.

[25] Dumoulin, C., E.J. Hay-Smith, and G. Mac Habee-Seguin, Pelvic floor muscle training versus no treatment, or inactive control treatments, for urinary incontinence in women. *Cochrane Database Syst. Rev.*, 2014(5): p. CD005654.

[26] Beyar, N. and A. Groutz, Pelvic floor muscle training for female stress urinary incontinence: Five years outcomes. *Neurourol. Urodyn.*, 2015.

[27] Bo, K., B. Kvarstein, and I. Nygaard, Lower urinary tract symptoms and pelvic floor muscle exercise adherence after 15 years. *Obstet. Gynecol.*, 2005. 105(5 Pt 1): p. 999-1005.

[28] Sherburn, M., et al., Incontinence improves in older women after intensive pelvic floor muscle training: an assessor-blinded randomized controlled trial. *Neurourol. Urodyn.*, 2011. 30(3): p. 317-24.

[29] Hirakawa, T., et al., Randomized controlled trial of pelvic floor muscle training with or without biofeedback for urinary incontinence. *Int. Urogynecol. J.*, 2013. 24(8): p. 1347-54.

[30] Herderschee, R., et al., Feedback or biofeedback to augment pelvic floor muscle training for urinary incontinence in women. *Cochrane Database Syst. Rev.*, 2011(7): p. CD009252.

[31] Resnick, N.M., et al., What predicts and what mediates the response of urge urinary incontinence to biofeedback? *Neurourol. Urodyn.*, 2013. 32(5): p. 408-15.

[32] Peters, K.M., et al., Randomized trial of percutaneous tibial nerve stimulation versus extended-release tolterodine: results from the overactive bladder innovative therapy trial. *J. Urol.*, 2009. 182(3): p. 1055-61.

[33] MacDiarmid, S.A., et al., Long-term durability of percutaneous tibial nerve stimulation for the treatment of overactive bladder. *J. Urol.*, 2010. 183(1): p. 234-40.

[34] Peters, K.M., et al., Randomized trial of percutaneous tibial nerve stimulation versus Sham efficacy in the treatment of overactive bladder syndrome: results from the SUmiT trial. *J. Urol.*, 2010. 183(4): p. 1438-43.

[35] Levin, P.J., et al., The efficacy of posterior tibial nerve stimulation for the treatment of overactive bladder in women: a systematic review. *Int. Urogynecol. J.*, 2012. 23(11): p. 1591-7.

[36] Kabay, S., et al., The clinical and urodynamic results of a 3-month percutaneous posterior tibial nerve stimulation treatment in patients with multiple sclerosis-related neurogenic bladder dysfunction. *Neurourol. Urodyn.*, 2009. 28(8): p. 964-8.

[37] Canbaz Kabay, S., et al., Long term sustained therapeutic effects of percutaneous posterior tibial nerve stimulation treatment of neurogenic overactive bladder in multiple sclerosis patients: 12-months results. *Neurourol. Urodyn*, 2015.

[38] Kabay, S., et al., The Clinical and Urodynamic Results of Percutaneous Posterior Tibial Nerve Stimulation on Neurogenic Detrusor Overactivity in Patients With Parkinson's Disease. *Urology*, 2016. 87: p. 76-81.

[39] Chapple, C.R., et al., The effects of antimuscarinic treatments in overactive bladder: an update of a systematic review and meta-analysis. *Eur. Urol.*, 2008. 54(3): p. 543-62.

[40] Rai, B.P., et al., Anticholinergic drugs versus non-drug active therapies for non-neurogenic overactive bladder syndrome in adults. *Cochrane*

Database Syst. Rev., 2012. 12: p. CD003193.

[41] Buser, N., et al., Efficacy and adverse events of antimuscarinics for treating overactive bladder: network meta-analyses. *Eur. Urol.*, 2012. 62(6): p. 1040-60.

[42] Gray, S.L., et al., Cumulative use of strong anticholinergics and incident dementia: a prospective cohort study. *JAMA Intern. Med.*, 2015. 175(3): p. 401-7.

[43] Chancellor, M.B., et al., Blood-brain barrier permeation and efflux exclusion of anticholinergics used in the treatment of overactive bladder. *Drugs Aging*, 2012. 29(4): p. 259-73.

[44] Lee, R.T., M. Bamberger, and P. Ellsworth, Impact of mirabegron extended-release on the treatment of overactive bladder with urge urinary incontinence, urgency, and frequency. *Res. Rep. Urol.*, 2013. 5: p. 147-57.

[45] G, D.A., A. Maria Condino, and P. Calvi, Involvement of beta3-adrenoceptors in the inhibitory control of cholinergic activity in human bladder: Direct evidence by [(3)H]-acetylcholine release experiments in the isolated detrusor. *Eur. J. Pharmacol.*, 2015. 758: p. 115-22.

[46] Nitti, V.W., et al., Results of a randomized phase III trial of mirabegron in patients with overactive bladder. J Urol, 2013. 189(4): p. 1388-95.

[47] Chapple, C.R., et al., Mirabegron in overactive bladder: a review of efficacy, safety, and tolerability. *Neurourol. Urodyn.*, 2014. 33(1): p. 17-30.

[48] Chapple, C., et al., Efficacy of the beta3-adrenoceptor agonist mirabegron for the treatment of overactive bladder by severity of incontinence at baseline: a post hoc analysis of pooled data from three randomised phase 3 trials. *Eur. Urol.*, 2015. 67(1): p. 11-4.

[49] Cardozo, L., et al., Short- and long-term efficacy and safety of duloxetine in women with predominant stress urinary incontinence. *Curr. Med. Res. Opin.*, 2010. 26(2): p. 253-61.

[50] Vella, M., J. Duckett, and M. Basu, Duloxetine 1 year on: the long-term outcome of a cohort of women prescribed duloxetine. *Int. Urogynecol. J. Pelvic Floor Dysfunct.*, 2008. 19(7): p. 961-4.

[51] Bump, R.C., et al., Long-term efficacy of duloxetine in women with stress urinary incontinence. *BJU Int.*, 2008. 102(2): p. 214-8.

[52] Li, J., et al., The role of duloxetine in stress urinary incontinence: a systematic review and meta-analysis. *Int. Urol. Nephrol.*, 2013. 45(3): p. 679-86.

[53] Steers, W.D., et al., Duloxetine compared with placebo for treating

women with symptoms of overactive bladder. *BJU Int.*, 2007. 100(2): p. 337-45.

[54] Barnes, P.M., B. Bloom, and R.L. Nahin, Complementary and alternative medicine use among adults and children: United States, 2007. *Natl. Health Stat. Report*, 2008(12): p. 1-23.

[55] Moquin, B., et al., Complementary and alternative medicine (CAM). *Geriatr. Nurs.*, 2009. 30(3): p. 196-203.

[56] Tempest, H., et al., Acupuncture in urological practice--a survey of urologists in England. *Complement Ther. Med.*, 2011. 19(1): p. 27-31.

[57] Liu, B., et al., Effect of blinding with a new pragmatic placebo needle: a randomized controlled crossover study. *Medicine* (Baltimore), 2014. 93(27): p. e200.

[58] Xu, H., et al., A phase 1 clinical study on the efficacy of electroacupuncture for female patients with mild to moderate stress incontinence. *Chin. J. Trad. Chin. Med. Phar.*, 2014. 29(12): p. 3755-3758.

[59] Xu, H., et al., A Pilot Randomized Placebo Controlled Trial of Electroacupuncture for Women with Pure Stress Urinary Incontinence. *PLoS One*, 2016. 11(3): p. e0150821.

[60] Liu, Z., et al., The efficacy and safety of electroacupuncture for women with pure stress urinary incontinence: study protocol for a multicenter randomized controlled trial. *Trials*, 2013. 14: p. 315.

[61] Zhang, J., W. Cheng, and M. Cai, Effects of electroacupuncture on overactive bladder refractory to anticholinergics: a single-blind randomised controlled trial. *Acupunct. Med.*, 2015.

[62] Feng, Q., et al., Quantity-effect Relationship of Electroacupuncture for Urge Incontinence: A Multicenter Randomized Controlled Trial. *J. Acupunct. Tuina. Sci.*, 2012. 10(1): p. 49-53.

[63] Minassian, V.A., et al., Severity of urinary incontinence and effect on quality of life in women by incontinence type. *Obstet. Gynecol.*, 2013. 121(5): p. 1083-90.

[64] Khullar, V., L. Cardozo, and R. Dmochowski, Mixed incontinence: current evidence and future perspectives. *Neurourol. Urodyn.*, 2010. 29(4): p. 618-22.

[65] Jin, C., X. Zhou, and R. Pang, Effect of electro-acupuncture on mixed urinary incontinence. *J. Clin. Acupunct. Med.*, 2013. 29(6): p. 59-60.

[66] Jin, C., X. Zhou, and R. Pang, Effect of electroacupuncture combined with tolterodine on treating female mixed urinary incontinence. *J. Wound Ostomy Continence Nurs.*, 2014. 41(3): p. 268-72.

[67] Field, T., Massage therapy research review. Complement *Ther. Clin. Pract.*, 2014. 20(4): p. 224-9.

[68] Kassolik, K., et al., The effectiveness of massage in stress urinary incontinence-case study. *Rehabil. Nurs.,* 2013. 38(6): p. 306-14.

[69] Ripoll, E. and D. Mahowald, Hatha Yoga therapy management of urologic disorders. *World J. Urol.*, 2002. 20(5): p. 306-9.

[70] Tenfelde, S. and L.W. Janusek, Yoga: a biobehavioral approach to reduce symptom distress in women with urge urinary incontinence. *J. Altern. Complement Med.*, 2014. 20(10): p. 737-42.

[71] Huang, A.J., et al., A group-based yoga therapy intervention for urinary incontinence in women: a pilot randomized trial. *Female Pelvic. Med. Reconstr. Surg.*, 2014. 20(3): p. 147-54.

[72] Lo, T.S., et al., Effect of extracorporeal magnetic energy stimulation on bothersome lower urinary tract symptoms and quality of life in female patients with stress urinary incontinence and overactive bladder. *J. Obstet. Gynaecol. Res.*, 2013. 39(11): p. 1526-32.

INDEX